Praise for Your Vibrant Hea[

"This book is chocked full of vital, valuable information for living a long, healthy, vibrant life. It is literally a handbook for a healthy heart. It is easy to read and easy to apply. I highly recommend it."

—Jack Canfield
Co-creator of *Chicken Soup to Inspire the Body and Soul®*
www.jackcanfield.com

"This revolutionary book on heart health is the most complete study ever done to show you how to live longer, better, happier and more vibrantly than you ever thought possible."

—Brian Tracy
Best-selling author of *The Psychology of Achievement*
www.briantracy.com

"Read this special book! *Your Vibrant Heart* is about the heart and its higher potentials, but perhaps most importantly, it's from the heart. Dr. Cynthia shares her own journey of the heart, as well as the wisdom from the hundreds of patients she's worked with over the years. What I like most about the book is that it shows us the real inside-job of health, how to draw on the power of love to reinvent ourselves from the inside out."

—Gay Hendricks, Ph.D.
Author of *Conscious Loving* and *The Big Leap*
www.hendricks.com

"This book is a wonderful read about the mind-heart connection, written by a scientifically based cardiologist. Dr. Cynthia gives you the motivational tools to create a happier brain and a healthier heart. Doctor's orders: read it, do it, feel it."

—William Sears, M.D.
Author of *Prime-Time Health*
www.drsearswellnessinstitute.org

"Dr Cynthia Thaik is THE doctor to open your mind and your life to the ways and the means to REAL health in every area of life. I recommend you not only read her book, but that you take her 'prescriptions' for better living. It may actually save your life!"

—Bob Proctor
Best-selling author of *You Were Born Rich*
www.proctorgallagherinstitute.com

"In *Your Vibrant Heart*, a new voice in mind–body medicine, cardiologist Cynthia Thaik, M.D., integrates valuable medical knowledge, scientific facts, and holistic practices. She shows you how to integrate meditation, mindfulness, yoga, and self-awareness in a powerful program that brings forth inner peace, well-being, and the dynamic balance we call health. Bravo, Dr. Cynthia!"

—Joan Borysenko, Ph.D.
Author of *New York Times*–best seller *Minding the Body, Mending the Mind*
www.joanborysenko.com

"The principle of dualism in Chinese culture argues that if reflection takes place in the brain, intelligence—also referred to as *shen*—lies in one's heart. Thanks to her dual culture, Dr. Cynthia does a fantastic job presenting her holistic view on health throughout her captivating and well-documented book, which is made accessible with simple words: words that come from the heart."

—Tran Tien Chanh, M.D.
Author of *Ideal Protein... Because It's Your Life*
www.idealprotein.com

"In *Your Vibrant Heart*, Dr. Cynthia Thaik provides a comprehensive guide for optimal health and wellness in our complex, modern world. She draws upon her impressive medical education, solid science, years of medical practice, and her own transformational life experience to share with us the secrets of mind–body–spirit balance that is channeled through the human heart. Dr. Cynthia provides invaluable advice for each of us to follow on our own search for health, vitality, and joy. *Your Vibrant Heart* describes a visionary, holistic view of medicine as positive proactive wellness and not just reactive disease cure, including the importance of whole-food nutrition as a dietary foundation for a healthy, vibrant heart, body, and mind."

—John J. Blair
Senior Vice President, NSA Juice Plus+®
Board Chair of the Council for Responsible Nutrition
www.crnusa.org

"If you want a healthy and happy heart, you're going to LOVE *Your Vibrant Heart*! Dr. Cynthia Thaik combines the latest scientific breakthroughs in health and nutrition with cutting-edge insights to support your emotional and spiritual well-being. Thoroughly researched and profoundly practical, this book will guide you on the path to a healthy heart and a more love-filled life. Read it and thrive!"

—Ocean Robbins
CEO, The Food Revolution Network
Coauthor of *Voices of the Food Revolution*
www.foodrevolution.org

"Reflecting both professional and personal experience, Dr. Cynthia has written a book of health and heart tenets that will heal body, mind, and spirit. It is exciting to welcome Dr. Cynthia into the growing community of M.D.s who embrace the value of natural healing. *Your Vibrant Heart* is a book that belongs in the library of anyone interested in health and longevity."

—OrganicAngela
Founder of www.nut-and-berry.com

"Dr. Cynthia reveals with elegant simplicity the inseparable bond between the mind, body, and soul that directly affects your vibrant heart. The prescription she has written is one of love, and this book is a must-read for anyone interested in living their best life! She presents the material in a unique fashion; concepts and tools can easily be integrated into our lives. An important book for all my clients."

—**Kathryn Ford**
Life Mastery Consultant
www.kathrynford.com

"I have had the privilege to work with Dr. Cynthia for over ten years as a registered nurse and a licensed nurse practitioner. She is a Harvard-trained cardiologist with impeccable credentials and a highly acclaimed research and clinical background. Besides her 'book smarts,' her true magic is in her love, energy, and excitement at sharing her belief that all patients have within them the ability to transform their health and their lives. She believes in personal responsibility. She is realistic and encourages small but concrete steps to initiate change. She shares it all in *Your Vibrant Heart*. She is a great mentor, educator, and physician."

—**Doddie Wilson, R.N.**
Sherman Oaks, CA

"What if it were possible to heal your heart or enjoy vibrant health, vitality, and flexibility of body and mind? What if it were possible to age with ease, grace, purpose, and passion? What if it were possible to live a life you LOVE? *Your Vibrant Heart* shows you how. Read and apply the life-mastery tools in Dr. Cynthia's book. She is a true master healer who embodies the best of East and West, of science and spirituality, of true health and happiness."

—**Toby Needleman**
Positive Psychology Coach
www.tobyneedleman.lifemasteryinstitute.com

"Dr. Cynthia's *Your Vibrant Heart* is inclusive of not only medical issues, but also of themes related to celebrating life's purpose. The book serves as a quick reference and provides valuable and practical tips to implement immediately in the areas of nutrition, exercise, and stress. The book is written with unexpected humor and wit and is easy to digest and comprehend."

—**Joanne Badeaux**
Attorney
www.dedicatedlaw.com

"I've gone to Dr. Thaik for years, and the reason is simple; she's a brilliant scientist, but that is not all. What sets her apart is her attention to the rest of the 'machine.' She teaches nutrition and speaks to her patients on the power of emotional well-being. It is apparent that what she strives for is bringing all of the parts together for complete (heart) health. She shares all of her passion and knowledge in this well written book."

—**Leslye A. Gustat**
Producer/Writer/Patient

What Patients are Saying

"In *Your Vibrant Heart*, Dr. Thaik shares all of her knowledge and wisdom to her patients. I am living proof of the benefits of following her teachings. Prior to meeting Dr. Thaik, I was hospitalized for a cerebral aneurysm caused by high blood pressure. Within two months, I lost fifteen pounds! My blood pressure returned to normal. My spirit was rejuvenated, and she gave me courage to not give up. Thank you so much, Dr. Thaik, for giving ME back."

—Manasnati Tancharoen
Los Angeles, CA

"Dr. Cynthia has been my cardiologist for many years. In this book she shares her own transformational journey to inspire and motivate you. She has a wealth of medical knowledge and communicates in a manner that is easy to understand and apply to daily living. She offers an alternative to conventional pharmacologic therapy and gives a balanced opinion to health and healing. She helped me improved my blood pressure and my heart arrhythmia. I am forever grateful to her."

—Michael Yost
Valencia, CA

"Dr. Thaik has evolved professionally, emotionally, and spiritually over the past five years, and it is an inspiration to witness. Dr. Thaik has helped me more than any other physician. She truly cares about my physical, emotional, and spiritual health. She helped me become more aware of my bad habits and develop a better diet, fitness, and lifestyle. My general health has greatly improved, and I will always be grateful. I am happy to see her expand her influence beyond her patients through the writing of this wonderful book."

—Randy Eriksen
Glendale, CA

"While waiting for my appointment with Dr. Thaik for heart fluttering, I picked up a review copy of her book, *Your Vibrant Heart*. The index listed a section called 'Be Still My Heart.' This section was written for me! Dr. Thaik ran some tests and determined that my heart was healthy and that having some irregular heartbeats was actually normal. Dr. Thaik evaluates you, not just your heart. This book is a wealth of information that will help you understand your heart and why it functions as it does. I thank her for all of her insight."

—Cathy Wild
Canyon Country, CA

"After struggling with arrhythmias for years, I followed Dr. Thaik's recommendation and stopped eating meat and dairy and shifted to a plant based diet. Within three years, a twenty-four-hour heart monitor showed a decrease in irregular heartbeats from 30,000 to 107 beats. Dr. Thaik's expertise and support can be found within this book and will guide you in a new approach to health!"

—David Feiss
Westlake Village, CA

Dr. Cynthia's

YOUR
VIBRANT
HEART

*Restoring Health, Strength & Spirit
from the Body's Core*

CYNTHIA THAIK, M.D.
Harvard-Trained Cardiologist

FOREWORDS BY *Mary Morrissey and Bernie Siegel*, M.D.

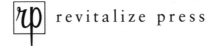 revitalize press

This book is intended as a reference volume only, not as a medical manual. The information given here is designed to help you make informed decisions about your health. It is not intended as a substitute for any treatment that may have been prescribed by your doctor. If you suspect that you have a medical problem, you should seek competent medical help. You should not begin a new health regimen without first consulting a medical professional. The names of individuals and the facts contained within the clinical histories have been altered to protect the privacy and identity of individuals and any resemblance to actual persons should be deemed coincidental.

Published by Revitalize Press, Burbank, CA
www.revitalizepress.com

Distributed by Greenleaf Book Group LLC
For ordering information, please contact Greenleaf BookGroup LLC at
P.O. Box 91869, Austin, TX 78709   ph. 512.891.6100
For special discounts for bulk purchases, please contact author at info@yourvibrantheart.com

Cover design by Peri Gabriel, www.knockoutbooks.com
Book design and layout by Mark Gelotte, www.markgelotte.com

Publisher's Cataloging-In-Publication Data
(Prepared by The Donohue Group, Inc.)

Thaik, Cynthia.
    Dr. Cynthia's Your vibrant heart : restoring health, strength & spirit
from the body's core / Cynthia Thaik. -- 1st ed.

    p. ; cm.

    Issued also as an ebook.
    Includes bibliographical references.
    ISBN: 978-0-9891041-2-8

    1. Heart--Diseases--Prevention. 2. Heart--Psychophysiology. 3.
Heart--Diseases--Alternative treatment. 4. Mind and body therapies. 5.
Alternative medicine. 6. Well-being. I. Title. II. Title: Your vibrant heart

RC682 .T43 2014
616.12   2013946626

Part of the Tree Neutral® program, which offsets the number of trees consumed in the production and printing of this book by taking proactive steps, such as planting trees in direct proportion to the number of trees used: www.treeneutral.com

Printed in the United States of America on acid-free paper

13 14 15 16 17 18   10 9 8 7 6 5 4 3 2 1

First Edition

TreeNeutral®

DEDICATION

To my children, Andrew, Sarah, and Jonathan Thein—you are my pride, my joy, my love.

To my husband, David Thein—thank you for all that you do for me; for loving me.

To my parents, Khin Su and Aung Thaik—your guidance and love made me who I am.

To my family—your love, encouragement, support, and patience made this book possible. You give me life, and you give me passion for my purpose.

Acknowledgements

I am so thankful for all the people who have contributed to the inspiration, creation, and success of this book. First and foremost, I want to give a shout of gratitude to the Universe and to all the spiritual people across the globe who have opened my eyes to new possibilities.

Thank you to the luminaries who were inspirations to me from the beginning: Sage Levine, Janet Attwood, Tama Kieves, Cynthia Kersey, Bob Proctor, Jack Canfield, and Michael Beckwith.

To my mentor, Mary Morrissey, and her Dream Builder team (www.marymorrissey.com), I am eternally grateful. I am also greatly indebted to Kimberly Micheli (www.oaktreecounseling.com) for her insight, wisdom, clarity, and friendship.

To my staff, I am so appreciative of all that you do for me. Thank you so much to Patrick, Doddie, Karla, Elizabeth, Lori, Brenda, Harriette, Shauna, and Bert. You are my second family.

To my book creation staff, this beautiful book is a testament to your professionalism. For their writing and research, thank you to the talented Deborah Jabbour and Stephanie Mee. I am grateful to my amazing editor, Helen Chang, and the team at Author Bridge Media (www.authorbridgemedia.com). For her strategic advice, thank you to Carol Abrahamson. Thank you to Peri Gabriel (www.knockoutbooks.com) and Mark Gelotte(www.markgelotte.com) for the beautiful cover design and the interior design and illustrations, respectively. I am grateful to my wonderful publicist, Marika Flatt, and her team (www.prbythebook.com), and to my media trainer, Ellie Scarborough Brett (www.mediabombshell.com). Thank you to Keith Richmond (www.facebook.com/PrinceOfTheGardenPoetry) for contributing the title. Lastly, thank you to Mary Morrissey and Dr. Bernie Siegel for their articulate and insightful forewords.

To my patients—you are my continuing education. Thank you for inspiring me to expand beyond my current knowledge so that I can offer you more paths to health and happiness.

Finally, to my family I owe the world. I am forever grateful to my parents, Khin Su and Aung Thaik. Your love, guidance, strength, and ethics have shaped me into the person that I am. To my brothers, Richard and Albert Thaik, I love you for all of my fond childhood memories. To my husband, David Thein, I am grateful to you for your love, for your sacrifices, and for being the bedrock of our family. To my son Jonathan, I live to watch you grow and embrace the gentle, kind, responsible young man that you have become. To Sarah, my beautiful daughter, you embody the teachings of this book, and your tenacity, ambition, and foresight will carry you far. To Andrew, my energetic, fun-loving free spirit, continue to imagine and create—you have only success in your future. To Jackie and Cecilia, my wonderful nannies, I could not have created this book without your help in taking care of my family. Thank you.

TABLE OF CONTENTS

FOREWORD

When the world was young, the gods upon Mount Olympus, having created the earth and man, the animals and the creatures of the sea, the trees and flowers and all living things, had one task remaining before them: they had to hide the secret of life. This secret was to remain elusive until man had evolved in consciousness to the point where he was ready to experience it.

The gods argued back and forth over where to conceal the secret of life. One said, "Let's hide it on the highest mountain. Man will never find it there."

A fellow deity replied, "We've created man with insatiable curiosity, ambition, and good strong legs. Eventually he will climb even the highest mountain."

Another god suggested burying the secret of life at the bottom of the deepest ocean. His cohorts sighed, "We created man with a burning desire to explore the world, and with a taste for seafood. Sooner or later, he will plumb even the greatest ocean depths."

Finally, one of the gods came up with a solution. "Let us hide the secret of life in the last place man will ever look, a place he will search only when he has exhausted every other possibility, and finally he is ready to discover it."

"And where is that?" asked the other gods.

To which the first god replied, "We will hide it deep in the human heart."

And so they did.

—Native American legend

Crushed by love, clogged by cholesterol, filled with joy, or squeezed by stress, the heart is the muscle of life itself. The condition of our heart defines who we are as human beings. We may be tender-hearted, jealous-hearted, lion-hearted, or chicken-hearted. An energetic octogenarian is young at heart; terrorists are downright heartless. Vulnerable people wear their hearts on their sleeves; Edgar Allen Poe's alter ego hid one beneath the floorboards.

The Bible contains an astonishing one thousand references to the heart, which still makes it a distant second to Hallmark. Bruce Springsteen had a hungry heart. Neil Young sought a heart of gold. While despair weighs heavily on the heart, hope makes it leap. True love compels us to give away our heart; thwarted romance makes us take it back again and guard the thing like Fort Knox. If compassion opens the heart, then bitterness can seal it off. Those who follow their hearts against all reason find greatness. Those who deny their hearts find happiness quite elusive.

Still, while telling people to "follow your heart" sounds inspiring, it leaves most of us floundering. We haven't a clue how to take the first step, much less move to the beat of our own hearts. If the heart readily identifies true love, then why do so many of us fall prey to its counterfeits? What magic ingredient opens a closed-down heart, enabling it to love again? What miracle renders a change of heart?

The heart has been an enigma that performs a complex, life-giving job every moment, yet we take its presence for granted until it literally breaks down—or just breaks.

> *"The heart has reasons that reason does not understand."*
> —Jacques Benigne Bossuel

No doubt about it, virtually every aspect of our lives involves the heart. Yet for all its prominence in literature and love songs, despite decades of medical research, this life force has remained a mystery until now, with the release of Dr. Cynthia Thaik's amazing book.

Your Vibrant Heart: Restoring Health, Strength & Spirit from the Body's Core is a powerful prescription for more joyful living that blends poignant stories of love with practical information about the role that emotions and daily choices play in heart health. Research shows that having a happy love life and supportive friends contributes greatly to heart health. Why, then, are people spending so much time being unhappy and alone?

I once read a story about Roberto De Vicenzo, the great Argentine golfer. A woman came to him in desperation after a tournament. Her baby was seriously ill, near death, she said, and she could not pay the doctor's bill. Perhaps he could spare just a tiny portion from some of his great earnings...? Touched by her plight, De Vicenzo gave the woman the money he'd just won in the tournament.

The next week, an official with the golf association contacted him. "I have news for you," the official said. "That woman has no sick baby. She doesn't even have a child. She fleeced you, my friend."

"You mean there is no baby who is dying?'" the golfer asked.

"That's right," confirmed the official.

"Then that's the best news I've heard all week," De Vicenzo replied.

How many of us would be so generous? What does it take to have a heart like De Vicenzo's?

In these pages, Dr. Cynthia answers the universal question, "What contributes to a generous, happy, and truly healthy heart?"

You are holding in your hands a once-in-a-lifetime book that offers a powerful healing path to anyone willing to stand up and begin the journey. Not only will your physical heart be better off for having experienced it; your entire life will be so, too.

These pages contain a treasure trove of keys to health and happiness. How you use them is entirely up to you. The only important thing is that you do use them. Because, as you are about to discover, this is not just a book you read. This is a book you live.

Mary Morrissey

Author, Speaker, Consultant
Building Your Field of Dreams
No Less than Greatness
www.MaryMorrissey.com

FOREWORD

The heart is a more significant part of our lives than most people are aware of. Its role is far more than to just provide us with a heartbeat and to circulate blood to our various organs. Think about how you feel when you speak about someone breaking your heart. Or just think about the increase in heart attacks that occur on Monday mornings. These things aren't coincidences, and there's a reason why that wonderful, therapeutic song tells us to let our hearts make up our minds.

As Dr. Cynthia Thaik shares in this book, when you have a vibrant heart, you are restoring your health from your inner core. Psyche and soma are no longer separate entities. They become a unit, working together to heal or to invoke illness.

It comes down to love. You have to love your life, and you have to love your body. When you feel that love within you, every organ will become vibrant, and health will flourish. Many studies have been done that prove this concept to be true. One example is Dr. Caroline Thomas, who studied and followed several medical students over many decades and, through their personality profiles and their drawings of the way they felt about themselves, found that she could predict which diseases they were going to get from that information and those symbols.

Another study done at Harvard showed that students who said they did not feel loved by their parents had an illness rate of nearly 100 percent by midlife. By contrast, those who felt loved only experienced a 25 percent rate of serious illnesses in the same period of time.

I have seen these same kinds of scenarios unfold in my practice. The body and our consciousness both speak through images, revealing psychic, somatic, and therapeutic information that cannot be known intellectually. Mind and body are a unit, and we must realize and accept that if we are to become responsible participants in our health and in our lives.

Built into each of us is the potential to induce healing through our internal chemistry—chemistry that is activated by our emotional life. I like to refer to this internal chemistry as our inner core. "Inner core" is an interesting term, because our life is literally stored in our bodies, as transplanted hearts and other organs have demonstrated.

By understanding and initiating our self-induced healing potential, we can lead our body's inner core down the path to restoring our health. Just as hunger leads us to seek nourishment, so can our problems and emotions lead us to the conclusion that we must nourish all aspects of our lives, which in turn has the power to activate our inner core's ability to heal.

What each of us must do is find meaning in our life and in the path we have chosen to follow. Too often, the catalyst for this kind of awakening comes in the form of a tragic event or illness that reminds us of the limited time we have on Earth. These events nevertheless become our turning points, and those who are willing to go within and learn from their difficulties are at last able to see life for the gift that it is.

Just as charcoal turns to diamond under pressure, the broken heart does more than simply heal: it becomes an energetic and vibrant source of life not only for the individual who possesses it, but for everyone around that person, as well. Achieving a healthy heart and spirit is a matter of finding harmony and rhythm in your life. You must love your life and your body, even when there are things going on that you don't like.

Learn to see yourself as a work of art that is always in the process of being created. You are continually reworking the canvas, and since it is always evolving, there is no sense in feeling like a failure at any point. Always remember to come back to love. To truly have a vibrant heart and a vibrant body, as well as a vibrant mind and a vibrant life, love must be present. Your body gives you the chance to demonstrate that love by living your authentic life. The life you choose to live may be the greatest of gifts or the most terrible of curses. The choice lies entirely in your hands.

What I ask of each of you is to become a warrior for love. You will fight with kindness, and tenderness will be your weapon of choice. You will be blind to the faults of others because love is blind, and you will love unconditionally with no expectations. When you do this, your energy field will change. Your heart will radiate its vibrancy to the benefit of all who you come into contact with. When we choose to enhance our own lives with love, we enhance the lives of others, as well.

So please, become a warrior for love. When you have succeeded in achieving health and fulfillment in your own life, become a life coach for others. Ours is a team that needs your contribution. A perfect world does not create itself. It is created out of love by the collective efforts of those who have developed a vibrant heart.

BERNIE SIEGEL, M.D.

Author of twelve books, including *Love, Medicine & Miracles*
www.BernieSiegelMD.com

INTRODUCTION

"You cannot solve a problem from the same consciousness that created it. You must learn to see the world anew."

—Albert Einstein

Life Is a Gift

Most people consider life to be their greatest gift. But for many, it is a gift that is not always created equal.

Although these individuals may have the gift of life—heart beating, blood circulating, lungs drawing air—without good health and a good heart, that gift is meaningless. If they are not able to run through a meadow, they cannot feel the gentle rush of the breeze on their skin. If they do not have the strength to hold their children in their arms, they cannot be warmed and comforted by that loving embrace. If their senses are impaired, they cannot enjoy the rich spectrum of color that surrounds them, or hear the music of birdsong.

Without a good heart, their paths through life are not a fascinating voyage of discovery and adventure. Instead, those paths become an endless and painful uphill

Life is a gift, and good health and a good heart should be our most prized possessions.

struggle for survival. Life is a gift, and good health and a good heart should be our most prized possessions.

The heart is the essence of our being and of our existence. Yet all too often, we fail to pay attention to it until the benefits that it bestows on us are taken from our grasp. This is a mistake that comes with terrible consequences. For when we examine our lives and the priorities that we place on our routines—careers, finances, relationships, successes, and failures—none of them carry much importance if we do not have our health as a base to support everything else.

Our health is a dynamic process, forever changing as we transition from periods of good health to moments of sickness and back again. Universally, our goal in achieving optimal health and wellness is this: to strive to continually improve the quality of our lives, our sense of well-being, our energy levels, and our mental capacities.

When approaching this far-reaching goal for the first time, many people do not know where to start—and understandably so. Thankfully, there are two clear and simple starting points: mindfulness and personal responsibility. These concepts, though underused, are not new. Mindfulness is the seventh element of the noble eightfold path to enlightenment, according to the teachings of the Buddha. When coupled with personal responsibility, all the actions necessary to attain optimum health can be achieved.

How do we define mindfulness? Mindfulness is the ability to gently focus a calm awareness on the current moment, allowing us to notice our present state in a nonjudgmental manner. Being mindful, and then accepting responsibility for the facts that our mindfulness reveals about us, frees us from the guilt, blame, and self-judgment of our past, as well as from the fears we hold about the future. Research has shown that practicing mindfulness is one of the most important skills for achieving a rapid awakening and an unconditional sense of fulfillment.

Yet far too many people fail to engage in the daily, deliberate acts that are needed to achieve this sense of well-being. They only desire good health once it is gone. Or if they have good health, they do not value it, placing health maintenance low on their priority lists. They do not appreciate the gift that they possess, and so they do not really value life itself.

> The life you desire, the health you desire, and the quality of your heart and your body are first created within your mind's eye.

It therefore behooves each of us to ask ourselves: What are my priorities when it comes to good health? Is health something I have, or is it something I desperately want?

Health and a vibrant, vivacious heart are not wholly physical things. The life you desire, the health you desire, and the quality of your heart and your body—both on a physical and on a metaphysical plane—are first created within your mind's eye. Yet far too many people are unaware of this, or they fail to utilize this gift to its fullest potential.

To be clear, having the power to visualize and to manifest the health and the heart you desire does not mean that you control your health mentally. It means that you are in control of the decisions that determine whether you can attain and maintain a strong heart. Training your mind to make your health and your heart a priority will change your life. You can and you will find the necessary balance between heart, body, mind, and soul. It's all up to you. You have the power to choose this path, and to create the heart of your dreams.

My Authentic Life

It's sometimes hard for me to believe how unfulfilling my world used to be. After I made the choice to pursue the path I have just described, my life transformed completely. In the span of two short years, it blossomed into something richer and more authentic than I ever thought was possible. I rediscovered my professional calling, and the spiritual path I traveled not only gave direction to my life, but also filled it with joy, hope, and wonderment at all the possibilities available to me.

Professionally, I became a doctor who delivered wellness and health, rather than one who just dealt with disease. Within the first two years of launching my wellness center, I orchestrated more beneficial outcomes for my patients than I had in all the preceding twenty years of practicing solely conventional medicine—several of which have been recorded in these pages, though names and some details have been changed for privacy. In essence, I became a true heart doctor: one who practiced with her heart, and one who valued life to its purest core.

This book reflects my transformation from a Harvard-trained cardiologist who practiced exclusively modern, conventional Western medicine to a better-rounded physician with a holistic practice that incorporates mindfulness, Eastern philosophy, and the mind-body-soul connection into health, and into life as a whole.

Hearkening Back: East Meets West

My earliest exposure to medicine came from my Eastern roots. I have vivid memories of accompanying my mother to her clinic in my home country, Myanmar, formerly known as Burma, when I was five years old. There, I saw patients windmill in and out, their ailments ranging from minor cuts and injuries to serious infections and internal organ issues.

My mother was a government employee, so there was no insurance or bureaucracy to deal with, and no direct exchange of money between her and her patients ever took place. She certainly had no concerns about malpractice allegations or lawsuits. It was just her and her patients, and both parties were always focused on the simple act of healing.

Years later, I—like my mother—made the decision to become a doctor. Two events in particular pushed me toward cardiology. The first was the opportunity to hold a living, beating heart during my residency—something that thrilled me even more than I had imagined it would.

The second was an experience I had with a young mother of two who had just been diagnosed with a malignant pericardial effusion, meaning that she had blood around her heart from newly diagnosed breast cancer. I was on duty when, that evening, she went into full cardiopulmonary arrest in the ICU room. After thirty minutes of trying to resuscitate her, just before pronouncing her dead, I, in a moment bursting with inspiration and desperation at once, decided to push a needle into her chest and connect it to a suction bottle. Incredibly, it worked, and her pulse and blood pressure (BP) returned. There was no feeling so daunting and yet so exhilarating—and no knowledge so humbling—as the realization that I had saved that woman's life.

From these roots, my career in cardiology was born. More than twenty years of practice followed, first in the academic settings of the Beth Israel Hospital and the Brigham and Women's Hospital in Boston, then at the University of California, Los Angeles Medical Center, and finally in private practice.

At first, I relished the opportunity to intersect with and impact so many lives. But over time, things began to change. My excitement for cardiology was replaced by the mundaneness of daily practice. A frustration began to grow in me—one that came from watching people fail to treasure the gift of life day in and day out.

It was the prelude to a remarkable change.

Personal Journey

By my fourteenth year of working as a cardiologist, my life was on the brink of collapse. The contractor in charge of building our new house not only abandoned the project in its final year, but also initiated litigation proceedings that cost us hundreds of thousands of dollars. Frustrations from that and from other things meant that relations with my husband were at a breaking point. I was becoming increasingly detached from my three children. I operated from day to day like a robot—with extreme efficiency, but little feeling. I felt numb inside.

The final straw came one day after a particularly bitter phone call from my husband left me reeling emotionally. That night, I went out to dinner with a friend, who gave me the phone number of a therapist named Kimberly Micheli. I knew that I had two choices: to call the therapist, or to stand by and watch my marriage splinter apart. A decision was in my hands that would change my life forever.

I chose to call the therapist.

For four months, Kimberly and I worked one-on-one together. She succeeded in finally pulling me out of my black hole and setting me on the right track. She was the one who first pointed out to me the simple truth: I was operating from the standpoint of being "all in my head."

That realization sent me reeling. For years, I had been following other people's rules. I had put myself entirely at the service first of my parents, then of my husband and my children. At no point in all those years had there been any time to take care of myself. In order to cope with that hard reality, I had trained myself to operate from the neck up. For a heart doctor, I had become drastically out of touch with my own heart.

Once I realized these things, there was no going back. I made the choice to start walking a new path—one of mindfulness and personal responsibility. Sure enough, under Kimberly's guidance, my life began to change. I started practicing yoga and meditation, and I committed myself to new habits of good nutrition and exercise.

The results were so impactful that they broke every expectation that my imagination had come to the table with. The more my mindfulness and personal responsibility grew, the faster positive changes began to take place.

Spurred by my success, I made the decision to start my wellness center. There, for the first time, I began talking to people not about their diseases, but about their health. Around this time, I also met my second mentor, Mary Morrissey, who became my life coach. Mary's philosophy is that you can do, achieve, or be anything that you want to be as long as you are committed to doing one thing: creating your vision. Her teachings pushed me to take my personal growth to the next level.

Before I knew it, my attitude and my approach to my patients had completely transformed. My cardiology practice and my wellness center had become hubs of fun, energy, and passion for me. It dawned on me that, in reformulating the way I practiced, I had at last discovered my divine purpose.

From that moment onward, everything was different. My relationship with my husband became one of love and respect. I stopped pushing my children to go-go-go all the time. Instead, I began feeding them healthier foods, and I started taking them to yoga with me. They are the only three children in our yoga class, and they enjoy it almost as much as I do. Our family atmosphere has become one of love and harmony.

This new me understands how to express herself in her own voice. She has learned how to manifest her authenticity, her spirit, and her joy. I feel strong, and I am secure in the knowledge that I am not alone. The universe is the source of my guidance, and my voice echoes its fundamental truth.

A New Path

In the end, my journey taught me the importance of pushing beyond the boundaries of my own box. It taught me to follow my own calling. That new goal became embodied in exploring the power of nutrition and starting my wellness clinic. It was a bold move, to say the least. I was convinced that it was up to me to draw my own path to fulfillment. That was exactly what I did.

Amidst a still high-paced, functional existence, I have created a life I love—one that is filled with peace, tranquility, and gratitude for all that I have and for all that I am. In the nine months after achieving my transformation, I took on more than I ever had before. I wrote this book. I built a national brand (www.drcynthia.com). I started a nonprofit organization, Revitalize Youth (www.revitalizeyouth.org). I began a speaking career. All the while, I ran two successful businesses.

In earlier years, that kind of schedule would have driven me into the ground. Yet I felt—and continue to feel—calm and at peace with my soul. My trust in the universe is profound, and I know that it will deliver what I need to make things work. This trust has been amply rewarded by the opportunities that have arisen to support my new success.

For instance, the first patient to whom I had the opportunity to announce my plan to write this book happened to be an English professor and a former editor. I have crossed paths with many others who have advanced my goals. I am a shining example of the Universal Law of Attraction at work. I am proof of the fact that you call into your life all that you set your intentions on.

Finally, on still another level, my spirituality blossomed in step with my emotional growth. Although I was raised as a Buddhist, I had lost touch with that element of my life during my "dark days." My transformation reconnected me with my childhood affinity with "God." The reemergence

---

QR Codes (black square module shown above) are provided throughout this book to link to websites. Using a smartphone, scan the code by holding the phone camera over the code until it reads the location. The scan will automatically go to the website. iPhones will need a QRreader app. The URLs have been provided for those without this capability.

of my spiritual faith played a strong role in allowing me to reflect on my professional life, as well. It was my rediscovered spirituality that put me in touch with my divine calling—the life purpose or mission that I was placed on this planet to complete.

These concepts of mindfulness, personal growth, and spirituality hold unimaginable power.

The knowledge feels real and magical at the same time, and it resonates with my entire being.

The Mind-Body Connection

These concepts of mindfulness, personal growth, and spirituality hold unimaginable power. Yet many people live their lives without ever discovering them, even though they are vital to our physical and spiritual health.

The mind-body connection is unparalleled in importance. Most, if not all, diseases (dis "ease") occur as a result of the misalignment of this mind-body axis. When there is an incongruence or disconnect in your life, and when you are not aligned with your inner guide, you become toxic to yourself. Not only do your emotions talk to you in the form of anxiety or depression, but your body also talks to you in the form of physical ailments. Gastrointestinal symptoms, chest pain, and palpitations are just a few signs of this imbalance.

To remedy this, we must learn to reconnect our bodies with our minds. We must learn the language in which our inner guide speaks to us. Every thought and every emotion leads to an instantaneous release of hundreds if not thousands of neurotransmitters within the brain and the body. Emotions affect every cell in the body through these neurotransmitters, either positively or negatively. New science is revealing that how you *respond* to your environment or to your circumstances can change your fate.

> When there is an incongruence or disconnect in your life, and when you are not aligned with your inner guide, you become toxic to yourself.

While this concept sounds simplistic, actually applying it in our daily lives is a much more challenging task. Even though we can control our conscious thoughts, an enormous part of our lives is dictated by our subconscious minds. Dr. Bruce Lipton proposes in his book *The Biology of Belief: Unleashing the Power of Consciousness* that our conscious mind is in charge 5 percent of the time, whereas our subconscious mind is in control 95 percent of the time. Much of our subconscious programming occurs during early childhood. Consequently, changing our lives into what we wish them to be truly requires a systematic, conscious reprogramming of our subconscious minds.

If we are to change our priorities and value our hearts and our health, then we need to make a conscientious effort to slow down the pace of our lives and to introduce pleasure, fun, serenity, and excitement into our daily activities. While the physical body's symptoms are important, if we are to achieve optimal health, we need to take care of our mental health and maintain the delicate balance of peace and harmony that exists between our mind and our body. We can reinvigorate our minds and create a higher vibratory energy through practices such as meditation, hypnosis, emotional freedom therapy or tapping, and brainwave entrainment to support our health.

Learning to develop mindfulness and to connect with your inner guide takes time, patience, and trust. You need to make the decision that there are certain things you know without being able to see, and that you need to trust in their existence. This decision is the beginning of healing. As a physician who has experienced this journey firsthand, I give my patients a glimpse of the possibilities available to them, and I expand their knowledge as well as their realities.

Patients often go to the doctor thinking that he or she will have the answers, plain and simple. But the truth is that patients themselves have a better chance of influencing their health than any doctor does. Many medical doctors are not willing to go deeper into the emotional or mental states of their patients, as I have learned to do with mine. My guidance is my gift to those who seek me out. Nevertheless, in the end, it is the patient who makes the choice to open his or her heart, mind, body, and soul to the possibility of reclaiming lost health.

This book is for those who are ready to take that step.

Proactive Change

Your Vibrant Heart: Restoring Health, Strength & Spirit from the Body's Core will reveal a world of possibilities to you on your journey toward achieving optimal health and a strong heart. The heart is an organ that does so much more than pump blood and sustain life. Your heart signifies energy, vibrancy, life, love, hope, happiness, vitality, strength, and spirit.

Achieving and maintaining a vibrant heart is not a passive task. You need to be proactive—not reactive—in order to end up where you aim to go. This book will guide you through that process by helping you to create a purposeful vision of the life and the health that you would love to have. It will show you how to align the physical, mental, and spiritual aspects of yourself in order to achieve your goal. The tool you need to take purposeful action is in your hands.

This book aims to shift the medical community's current paradigm of a symptom- and disease-based model of practice. As a practicing cardiologist, it is my goal to change that paradigm into one that fosters and actively promotes wellness. I want patients to see their health-care

Your heart signifies energy, vibrancy, life, love, hope, happiness, vitality, strength, and spirit.

providers for wellness checks rather than for symptoms or for managing existing diseases. It is my hope that my colleagues will be inspired by this book's teachings to increase their awareness of the potential of the mind to supplement their work of healing.

As physicians, it falls to us to be the teachers of this awesome potential of life, and to awaken in our patients the knowledge that they can guide their own process of healing and of being. We have the task and the privilege of informing them of the vast options and resources that are available to calm their fears and concerns, improve their mindfulness, and change their outlooks on their cardiac symptoms and on their health as a whole.

For individuals in search of healing, the tools for change are at your fingertips. You have only to reach out and seize them. Interwoven throughout these chapters is the concept of "brave thinking." According to Mary Morrissey, "Brave thinking requires a strategy of navigating the mind to think in a manner that is generative rather than contractive." All too often, we let our circumstances dictate our moods, our thoughts, and our actions. We let life control us, rather than taking control of our lives.

Brave thinking allows us to change the frequency of our vibrational energy and, consequently, the circumstances in which we exist. It allows us to leave behind fear and self-doubt. Most of all, it allows for increased self-awareness, which ultimately lies at the root of health. Brave thinking is the catalyst that each of us requires to put ourselves on the path to good health.

The true power of healing—of making our beings whole—exists in each and every one of us. By nature, we are meant to be healthy. Your body, mind, spirit, and soul will move you into a state of health all on their own, as long as you are willing to create the opportunity for them to do so.

> Brave thinking requires a strategy of navigating the mind to think in a manner that is generative rather than contractive.

Health in Bloom

The new path to health blends modern medicine with Eastern philosophies. It delivers knowledge through education. It emphasizes personal responsibility, mindfulness, and higher consciousness, and it

The true power of healing—of making our beings whole—exists in each and every one of us.

provides support through health and life coaching. By following this path, I have made huge differences in my patients' health and lives, and I have brought joy and fulfillment back into my own life, as well.

This book celebrates the magnificence of our exquisite hearts and pays tribute to the miracle of creation of this splendid organ. It explores the role of the heart as the essence of life, providing and sustaining us with meaning, emotion, and the spirit of existence. Although it covers the topics of the physical heart, it also emphasizes different aspects of life—such as love, laughter, and awareness—that are equally important to achieving heart health.

We have all been given the gift of life. If you respect that gift by treating good health and a strong heart as your most precious possessions, you will experience life to the fullest. A vibrant heart is within your grasp. You have the power to reach out your hand and embrace it. The time has come to change your perception of life, to increase your vibratory energy, and to define and create your unique vision. When you do, an empowered and uplifted heart will follow.

I invite you to join me on the journey of a lifetime—a journey that will transform your life, renew your health, and revitalize your heart, your mind, your body, and your spirit. Together, we will attain what we all desire: a life filled with peace, energy, love, joy, and well-being. To your health! To Your Vibrant Heart!

CHAPTER 1

THE HEART IS A MANY-SPLENDORED THING

"What is straight? A line can be straight, or a street, but the human heart, oh, no; it's curved like a road through mountains."

—Tennessee Williams

What Is a Heart?

When the Four Aces sang "Love Is a Many-Splendored Thing," they were inadvertently referring to a complex set of emotions triggered by the heart. The lyrics would not have been quite as catchy if "love" was replaced with "heart." Yet in reality, it is the heart itself that is a thing of splendor—an incredibly complex, unmatched work of art with multiple facets, each as magnificent as the other.

I am not referring just to the marvel of the physical heart, but also to the metaphysical heart—the heart that not only keeps us alive, but represents the different aspects of self: emotions, mind, body, soul, and spirit.

The heart has long been recognized as a symbol of love, but it is also referred to

The heart has long been recognized as a symbol of love, but it is also referred to as the spiritual, emotional, moral, and even intellectual core of the human body.

as the spiritual, emotional, moral, and even intellectual core of the human body. The heart was once believed to be the seat of the human soul. In various religions, the heart symbol also has numerous meanings, including charity, hope, energy, flow, happiness, and joy.

In this chapter, we will explore the facets of your physical and spiritual heart. We'll begin at what most people perceive to be the beginning: the physical heart and where it comes from.

STAGES OF HEART DEVELOPMENT

While we might debate for ages about whether life starts at the point of conception, there is no arguing that life is present in the first heartbeat, which occurs approximately twenty-one days after conception.

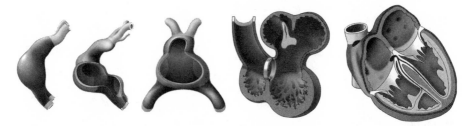

Fig. 1-1   Stages of Heart Development

As seen in Figure 1-1, heart development has five stages. It begins when cardiac precursor cells migrate to form a primitive heart tube. Even at the very early stage as a tube, the heart has different regions and layers. The primitive heart tube closely resembles a fish heart, and it is within this tube that the first flickering of a heartbeat is detected.

In the second stage of heart development, called heart looping, the tube-shaped heart contours into an S shape, bending to the right in a d-looping. It is within this contour that the chambers of the heart will develop.

The third stage, called the two-chambered stage, allows for the development of the two-chambered (one atrium, one ventricle) heart, which resembles the heart of a frog.

The fourth stage of development is the three-chambered heart, triggered by the atrium dividing into two atria. At this stage, the embryo heart resembles that of a snake or a turtle heart.

The final stage of heart development occurs by the end of the tenth week of pregnancy, with the development of the four-chambered heart consisting of two atria, two ventricles, and two great blood vessels—distinguished as a human heart and capable of running a fully functional cardiovascular system.

Given the complexities and intricacies of heart development, it is amazing that in most live births the heart is perfectly formed and functional.

Similarly, it is of no surprise that heart defects are the most common type of birth defect in the United States, affecting nearly 1 percent of births a year (approximately forty thousand births). Heart defect is the leading cause of birth-defect-related illness or death. It is estimated that 15 percent of heart defects are associated with a genetic condition. Approximately 20 to 30 percent of those with heart defects have other physical, developmental, or cognitive problems.

Today, the prevalence of minor cardiac defects is increasing, while the prevalence of more serious defects is stable. The survival rates of the more serious cardiac defects have significantly improved with better diagnostic tools and surgical treatment.

Given the complexities and intricacies of heart development, it is amazing that in most live births the heart is perfectly formed and functional.

Based on available studies, the federal Centers for Disease Control and Prevention (CDC), based in Atlanta, estimates that more than one million adults in the United States live with a heart defect. Most of these people survive into adulthood, and while there might be some limitation to exercise capacity, most live normal or near-normal lives.

How Your Physical Heart Works

The primary function of a heart is to deliver oxygen-rich blood to the cells and organs of the body. Each person's magnificent heart functions tirelessly, beating approximately 80,000 to 140,000 times a day, depending on the resting heart rate. This accounts for forty-two million heartbeats a year. An average resting cardiac output would be 5.6 liters per minute for a human male and 4.9 liters per minute for a female, but the heart is capable of delivering three to four times that amount during exercise, and a world-class athlete can deliver up to 40 liters per minute.

The blood circulates in a closed-circuit system, returning to the heart from the rest of the body through the venous system of blood vessels. The blood travels through the right atrium through the tricuspid valve into the right ventricle. From there, it travels through the pulmonary valve into the pulmonary vessels, traversing the lung alveoli, picking up oxygen for the blood cells. From the lung, the blood travels back through the left atrium through the mitral valve into the left ventricle.

The left ventricle is considered the main workhorse of the heart. It is the chamber responsible for propelling the blood through the aortic valve to the rest of the body through arterial blood vessel circulation. Figure 1-2 demonstrates the path of blood flow through the heart.

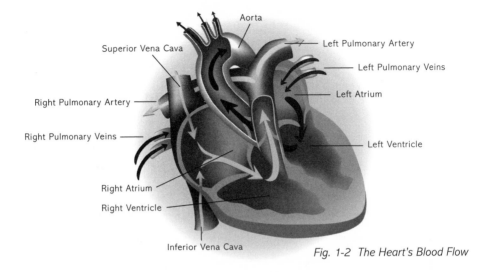

Aorta

Superior Vena Cava

Left Pulmonary Artery

Left Pulmonary Veins

Left Atrium

Right Pulmonary Artery

Right Pulmonary Veins

Left Ventricle

Right Atrium

Right Ventricle

Inferior Vena Cava

Fig. 1-2 The Heart's Blood Flow

THE AMAZING WORK OF CARDIAC CELLS

There is no reliable scientific knowledge of the number of cells comprising the human heart, although one abstract hypothesis estimates, using DNA content measurement, that there are hundreds of millions to billions of cardiac cells.

It was once thought that neither the human heart cells nor the brain cells were capable of regenerating, but we now know otherwise. Scientists from the Karolinska Institute in Sweden report that into early adulthood, we're continually renewing about 1 percent of our heart cells a year. That regeneration slows down, but it still occurs in old age, with a little less than half of 1 percent of cells regenerating at age seventy-five. All told, we've renewed about 40 percent of our heart cells by age seventy, neuro-scientist Jonas Frisén told *Science* magazine, providing hope that even a damaged heart stands a chance of being repaired to health.

Regardless of the number of cardiac cells, the cells of the heart work together as a functional syncytium—with all the cardiac muscle cells interconnected to one another mechanically, chemically, and electrically, and acting as a single enormous muscle.

PHYSICAL HEART, EMOTIONAL HEART

The connection between the physical heart and the emotional heart can be expressed in any number of ways. For me, one of the most stirring expressions of it comes through the miracle of motherhood. In comparison to what I experienced twenty-five years ago in my training, the advances of modern technology now allow physicians to diagnose many complex congenital heart diseases and even intervene in utero.

A MOTHER'S FAITH

Kari, a pharmaceutical representative who visits me often, was at age thirty-seven excitedly anticipating the birth of her second child. All blood tests required by the state showed her chances of having a baby with any birth defect to be low.

Then, out of the blue, the unthinkable showed up at her seventh-month ultrasound. Her baby was found to have transposition of the great arteries: there was no crossing of the baby's blood from the right to the left side of the organ.

Kari's heart sank as she was told that her baby did not have a chance of surviving and that she should consider an abortion. The next week brought a frantic pace of repeat ultrasounds, as well as consultations with four pediatric cardiologists and one of the top cardiothoracic surgeons in the area.

The decision to keep her child was based in faith. Her son's open-heart surgery on his third day of life lasted three-and-a-half hours. Today he is a beautiful three-year-old boy in great shape, and other than the scar on his chest, you would not know that he was born with a life-threatening heart defect.

Unfortunately, not all of these stories have happy endings. After feeling the exhilaration and utter joy of having given birth to a perfectly formed and healthy baby boy, Jonathan, I experienced two miscarriages in quick succession. My second conception resulted in a pregnancy that did not reveal a heartbeat in the expected third or fourth week. Yet even the sadness and disappointment of that loss pales in comparison to the experience of our third child, who survived several weeks longer.

Any mother who has undergone such a loss understands the fear and anticipation of the first ultrasound scanning for any detection of the heartbeat that signifies life. To have felt the comfort and relief of seeing a heart beating at the appropriate heart rate at the third week, only to have a repeat ultrasound two weeks later reveal a still heart, created a pain beyond belief.

Even though both children died early in their development, the emotions I experienced after their losses were devastating. The magnitude of the second loss was intensified by the mere presence of a heartbeat for a few short weeks.

I can only imagine, then, the pain when the loss occurs just minutes or hours or days after a full birth. I witnessed the intense sorrow of a young mother who held her newborn boy for just a few short hours after he was born with a multitude of congenital defects (including cardiac), which were well beyond any remedy that modern medicine could offer at that time.

As the young mother gently caressed that child, kissing, hugging, and holding him in her arms, I—a young medical student not yet having undergone my own tragedies—wondered which would be a worse fate: to have a few short hours of being able to hold that breathing, living, warm being and to feel and hear that heartbeat before losing the child, or to lose the child within the womb and never have the child be born alive at all.

Anyone who has experienced motherhood knows the myriad emotions that one experiences upon learning that within your body lives the heartbeat of another. The nine months of incubation allow for a full appreciation of the awesomeness of creation. This being, who started from the division of a single cell, develops complex nerve connections, digestive organs, and functioning cardiac, circulatory, and other systems—all within nine short months.

One can truly appreciate the marvels of creation when one considers that only a very small percentage of live births result in a baby not being anatomically perfect with ten fingers, ten toes, and a beautifully formed face with all of its components. Those of us who have had the misfortune of experiencing otherwise also have a great appreciation for the delicacies of this process. Fortunately for me, the universe rewards patience and persistence. My faith in the miracle of life was restored following the births of my beautiful daughter, Sarah, and my energetic boy, Andrew.

THE EMOTIONAL HEART

The intricacies and the complexities of the physical heart are paralleled by the intricacies and complexities of the emotional heart. Many would argue, and appropriately so, that navigating through life with the emotional heart is like maneuvering through a labyrinth marked by temperamental swings from deep despair to heights of exhilaration.

Navigating through life with the emotional heart is like maneuvering through a labyrinth marked by temperamental swings from deep despair to heights of exhilaration.

Unlike the physical heart that needs to deal only with physical stress, the emotional heart must deal not only with physical stress, but also with emotional, mental, and psychological stress. Whereas the physical heart only has to adapt to the makeup of the individual, the emotional heart deals with the rewards and burdens of self and is greatly influenced by interactions with loved ones, society at large, and the environment.

Emotion is energy in motion, and it represents the energy that flows from and through our heart to the rest of our body.

All too often, we tend to run away from our emotions, as if acknowledging their existence is a sign of weakness. But if we don't embrace and allow our emotions to express themselves, then their vibratory energy becomes internalized and becomes expressed in the form of symptoms, or dis "ease." Denying their existence does nothing to ease the pain, but rather prevents us from enjoying life as it is truly meant to be experienced.

Emotion is energy in motion, and it represents the energy that flows from and through our heart to the rest of our body. By embracing the emotions that flow from our heart, we harness the love, kindness, compassion, warmth, harmony, joy, peace, appreciation, gratitude, and resilience that reside in all of us.

AN EMOTIONAL HEART ATTACK

The heart is a symbol of love, and love is an emotion. All emotions vibrate at different frequencies. Anger, hatred, and resentment have low vibratory energies. Happiness, joy, and kindness have high ones. The emotions of love and gratitude vibrate at the highest frequency. Love heals the heart and inspires peace, harmony, and calmness. In order to maintain a balanced and healthy physical heart, we must take care to feed the emotional heart.

An emotionally broken heart has been shown to lead to a physically broken heart. Dr. Stephen T. Sinatra—a board-certified cardiologist and certified psychotherapist with forty years of clinical experience in treating, preventing, and reversing heart disease—in his book *Heartbreak and Heart Disease* speaks about this all-important mind-body connection to heart disease. It is estimated that 1 to 2 percent of patients diagnosed with a heart attack in the United States suffers from an emotionally broken heart. The presentation is very similar (chest pain, shortness of breath, palpitations), but the pathophysiology is markedly different.

A physical heart attack is usually caused by a blockage of the coronary artery by either atherosclerosis (the hardening of the blood vessel with cholesterol and other depositions) or thrombosis (blood clotting).

An emotional heart attack is caused by a surge of adrenaline and other neurohormones, which overwhelms and weakens the heart muscle, leading to a ballooning of the apex and causing the heart to take the shape of a Japanese teapot—thus its name, takotsubo cardiomyopathy ("tako-tsubo" means "fishing pot for trapping octopus"). It is also referred to as broken-heart syndrome.

While there are a few different artery anomalies among the proposed origins for broken-heart syndrome, case studies looking at the larger picture suggest that emotional triggers or clinical stressors (such as an asthma attack or a sudden illness) are often present. The prevalence is higher in the winter months, and the vast majority of the patients are female, typically postmenopausal.

I saw a case of broken-heart syndrome in my career. It was during a terrible snowstorm, when a mother and her teenage son were brought into the emergency room after a catastrophic automobile accident.

The mother had been driving and had suffered only minor cuts and injuries, while her son was severely injured. She was in near hysterics as she watched the emergency-room personnel work frantically to save her son's life.

Suddenly, she clutched her chest and slumped over. She was having a heart attack, but subsequent tests did not reveal any significant blockage of her arteries. The conclusion was that the extreme emotional stress of the automobile accident and the fear of her child's potential demise triggered the attack. Fortunately, both mother and son survived.

Although the above example is an extreme case, it is vital that we take care of our emotional health, as negative emotions have a tremendous impact on our heart and our overall health. Negative emotions often lead to despair and depression, which have been shown to wreak biological havoc within our bodies. Depression leads to the increased secretion of cortisol, a stress hormone released by the adrenal glands that is associated with heart disease, diabetes, and obesity.

Surges of neurotransmitters, such as serotonin and norepinephrine, can also lead to agitation, restlessness, anxiety, high blood pressure, and rapid heart rate. Depression also leads to increased inflammatory markers, such as C-Reactive Proteins (CRP), which have been shown to predict future heart-attack risk. Depression is furthermore linked to diminution of the immune system.

While these neurotransmitters, hormones, and other biochemical and physiological things are no doubt playing some role in heart disease and diabetes, a study from the VA Medical Center in San Francisco suggests that indirect factors, related to negative lifestyle choices made by the depressed person, hold even more sway.

It is a common emotion to feel sadness and depression following a heart attack, as the reality of the near-death experience and the vulnerability of life takes hold. However, remaining depressed can have a significant impact on the eventual outcome and prognosis of the individual.

In one landmark study, the continued presence of depression after recovery increased the risk of death to 17 percent within six months after a heart attack (versus 3 percent mortality in heart-attack patients who didn't have depression). That's the power of the emotional heart.

THE SPIRITUAL HEART

The spiritual heart or metaphysical heart takes the relationship to an even deeper level, connecting the mind, body, and spirit. Being aware or connected to your spiritual heart brings about a calm sense of inner peace and well-being. Spiritual practices such as meditation and prayer, as well as exercises such as yoga, tai chi, and qigong, often attempt to focus awareness on the spiritual heart center. At the core of our heart center is our true self.

When you allow yourself to listen to your heart and to trust your heart center, then you tap into the infinite wisdom of spiritual intelligence, which far supersedes your mind's intellect or your emotional judgment. While the mind tends to keep us ever present and constantly draws on logic to determine reality, the spiritual heart is free to dream and defy logic, and therefore it can create wonders that would not otherwise exist. It is with this belief that we can manifest our heart's desires.

Hridaya is a Sanskrit word meaning "this heart center." It is said to be different from the physical heart, and it is thought

> When you allow yourself to listen to your heart and to trust your heart center, then you are tapping into the infinite wisdom of spiritual intelligence, which far supersedes your mind's intellect or your emotional judgment.

to be located on the right side of the body. Ancient Asian cultures consider this heart center to be the seat of the soul. This spiritual heart is our ultimate connection to the universe. Through the practice of meditation, which focuses on the spiritual heart, we join in oneness, with one universal heart, one universal mind, and one universal consciousness. Knowledge and compassion are fundamental to this spiritual heart.

To better understand the nature of your spiritual heart, it helps to understand the nature of energy flow throughout your whole body.

According to ancient metaphysical tradition, seven major energy or psychic centers radiate throughout the body, called chakras. The word chakra means "energy disc" or "vortex." These seven energy stations are positioned from the base of the spine to the top of the head. Each plays a key role in regulating the body's vital life-force energy, known as "qi" in Chinese.

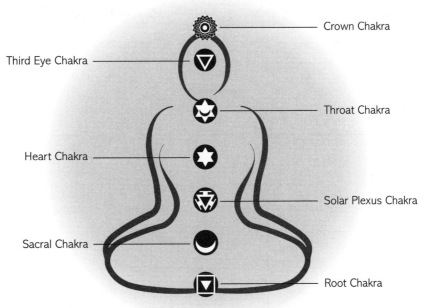

Crown Chakra

Third Eye Chakra

Throat Chakra

Heart Chakra

Solar Plexus Chakra

Sacral Chakra

Root Chakra

Fig. 1-3   The Chakras

The first chakra, Root, located at the base of the spine, is represented by red and the element of earth. It is the foundation of our physical body and influences our basic impulses for survival, including physical sensations and functions. It also strengthens our immune systems.

The second chakra, Sacral, located near the lower abdomen, is represented by the color orange and the element of water. It deals with sexuality and relationships and is the foundation of our emotional body.

The third chakra, Solar Plexus, located at the base of the rib cage, is represented by yellow and the element of fire. It is the foundation of our mental body, and it involves personal power, self-control, self-esteem, and self-acceptance.

The fourth chakra, Heart, located in the center of our chest, is represented by the color green and the element of air. It governs the

COLOR	CHAKRA	LOCATION	ELEMENT	FUNCTION/SYSTEM
Red	First / Root	Base of the spine	Earth	Grounding and survival
Orange	Second / Sacral	Lower abdomen, genitals	Water	Emotions, sexuality, relationships
Yellow	Third / Solar Plexus	Base of rib cage	Fire	Power, ego, self-control, self-esteem
Green	Fourth / Heart	Center of chest	Air	Love, sense of responsibility, forgiveness, self-acceptance
Blue	Fifth / Throat	Base of neck	Sound	Physical and spiritual communication, self-truth
Indigo	Sixth / Third Eye	Center of eyebrows	Light	Intuition, imagination, insight, enlightenment
Violet	Seventh / Crown	Top of head	Thought	Divine inspiration, guidance, connection to God or spirit

Fig. 1-4   Chakra System

heart, circulatory system, respiratory system, arms, shoulders, hands, diaphragm, ribs, breast, and thymus gland. This heart chakra is associated with unconditional love, self-acceptance, and forgiveness, and it brings with it tremendous healing power. The heart chakra is the foundation of the astral body, the connection between our physical body and our spiritual body. Learning to love oneself is the initial step in achieving a healthy heart chakra and becoming a healthy, balanced person.

The fifth chakra, Throat, located at the base of the neck, is represented by blue and the element of sound. It allows for communication and the expression of self-truth.

The sixth chakra, Third Eye, is positioned between the eyebrows and is represented by indigo and the element of light. It deals with intuition, imagination, insight, self-reflection, and enlightenment.

The seventh chakra, Crown, is represented by the color violet and the element of thought. It is located

MIND-BODY AXIS

THE POWER OF CHAKRAS

Many people disregard the chakras out of hand because they do not see the direct correlation between this energetic practice and the physical body. However, the truth is that the chakras and physical health are intimately connected. You can think of the chakras like spokes on a wheel. All the spokes need to be in working order for the wheel to turn. The same is true of the chakras: each of them needs to be balanced in order for energy to flow through the body in the healthy way that it is designed to do. When we have balanced chakras, it means that we have a balanced energy system, which contributes to our overall health.

However, we can also get more specific. Each chakra is associated with a specific part of the body, and their collective balance or lack thereof is consequently associated with the strength or the maladies that also take place in that part of the body. For example, the heart chakra is the center of love and tenderness, but it is also physically the center of blood and circulation. An imbalance of energy in the heart chakra could therefore cause a disease related to those physical things, not to mention emotional maladies such as emotional blocks. That is the link between the energetic chakras and our physical bodies, and it should never be underestimated.

at the top of the head and represents our connection to God or a higher spirit, divine inspiration, and guidance.

There are many factors that contribute to optimal heart health, and balance must be achieved so that the pieces will work in harmony.

Attention to the physical body is very important in terms of diet, exercise, and healthy lifestyle, but this will not maintain an overall healthy, happy heart if we neglect the emotional and spiritual aspects of the equation. Keep the emotional and spiritual heart healthy, and the physical heart will be healthy, too.

CHAPTER 2

THIS OLD HEART OF MINE

"When we long for life without difficulties, remind us that oaks grow strong in contrary winds and diamonds are made under pressure."

—Peter Marshall

The heart of the matter is: it is the heart that matters.

Do we value this vitally important, life-sustaining structure, or do we ignore its existence, neglecting its needs, devaluing its importance, and not recognizing its worth until it is too late? The real question here is this: Is your heart beating or ticking?

A heart that beats is sustaining life, providing vital circulation to the body, oxygenating each cell, and infusing each organ with strength. A heart that ticks is a time bomb waiting to explode, weighed down by stress, fear, anxiety, anger, and deadlines, and the list goes on. Answering this all-important question can mean the difference between life and death.

The maladies of the physical heart are numerous and dangerous. As with any undertaking, the key to good health starts with awareness. In this chapter, we will draw the big picture of the issues that the developed world is facing when it comes to physical heart health.

CARDIOVASCULAR DISEASE

Cardiovascular disease comprises different diseases that affect three main functions of the heart: blood flow or circulation, the mechanical function or the pump, and the electrical circuitry system.

CIRCULATION

The first component deals with blood flow directly to the heart muscle and systemically to the rest of the body. This can involve the accumulation of plaque within the blood vessels supplying the heart. Alternately, it can involve the blood vessels to the brain, mainly the carotid arteries and the intracranial blood vessels.

Finally, blood flow can also be an issue with the circulation of the peripheral vessels, mainly the abdominal aorta and the upper and lower extremities. Diseases that fall into the blood-flow category include coronary artery disease, cerebrovascular disease, and peripheral vascular disease.

Coronary Artery Disease

One of the leading causes of death in the United States having to do with blood flow to the heart is coronary artery disease.

According to statistics from 2009, more than 386,000 Americans died of heart disease that year, accounting for one out of six deaths in the country. Each year, approximately 635,000 Americans suffer their first coronary artery attack, and another 280,000 suffer multiple attacks. There are an additional 150,000 silent heart attacks annually. In 2010, coronary artery disease alone cost the United States more than $100 billion.

I like to call heart disease an equal-opportunity killer, affecting men and women equally. Despite this fact, as recently as 1997, only one in three women was aware that heart disease was their leading killer. This led the AHA to initiate an awareness effort culminating in the launch of the Go Red for Women campaign in 2003. The most recent study reported at the AHA meeting in 2013 showed that awareness of heart disease as the leading cause of women's death had nearly doubled from fifteen years earlier.

Coronary artery disease is signified by cholesterol-containing plaque building up in the arteries, which restricts blood flow. Evidence of this buildup—called atheroma—can occur in early childhood and even in utero in extreme cases where families have significant histories of high cholesterol.

While this atheromatous plaque is the most common sign of coronary artery disease, the narrowing of the inside of the blood vessels by the contraction of the muscle cells within the arterial walls (known as coronary vasospasm) and plaque rupture can also be the origin of heart attacks. Acute heart attacks are typically caused by a plaque rupture in lesions in the arteries that previously looked insignificant and did not cause discomfort. The slow progression of plaque can furthermore lead to chest pain (called angina).

Other common symptoms of coronary artery disease can include tightness or pressure in the chest, shortness of breath, and fatigue. The pain from these symptoms will occasionally radiate into the jaws, upper shoulders, and arms. In some cases—especially in women—individuals may experience feelings of sharp discomfort in the abdomen, back, and shoulder areas. Less common symptoms include palpitations, dizziness, sweating, nausea, and vomiting.

Unfortunately, symptoms do not always accompany the disease, which can make it particularly dangerous. Nor is coronary artery disease limited to those who are ill or more advanced in age. It can also cause acute heart attack or even sudden death in those who are young and who otherwise appear to be healthy. Tim Russert, the chief of NBC News's Washington bureau and the host of *Meet the Press*, possibly died in this manner in 2008.

One activity that has become associated with heart attacks is marathon running. The risk of dying while running a marathon is low (0.8 out of every 100,000 runners, according to a 2007 study published by the *British Medical Journal*), but a handful of race-related deaths do occur each year. Most of these are young people in the prime of life, under the age of forty.

In such cases, the culprit of the heart attack is less likely to be coronary artery disease. Rather, it is more likely to be related to increased inflammation of and decreased blood flow to the heart muscle, along with dehydration. Regardless of age or physical condition, it is always prudent to undergo a thorough physical and cardiovascular examination before engaging in any strenuous physical activity.

With coronary artery disease as with many other ailments, keeping track of personal risk factors—such as high blood pressure, high cholesterol, diabetes, family history, smoking, obesity, and physical inactivity—can be invaluable in preventing the illness.

While a host of medications and interventional procedures have been designed to address coronary artery plaquing, none of them have been shown to increase the rate of survival once the disease has developed. The ability to reverse heart disease lies instead within each individual who makes the decision to implement aggressive lifestyle modifications.

Books such as Dr. Dean Ornish's *Program for Reversing Heart Disease*, John McDougall's *The McDougall Program for a Healthy Heart*, Dr. Caldwell Esselstyn's *Prevent and Reverse Heart Disease*, Dr. Joel Fuhrman's *Eat to Live* and *Eat for Health*, and John Robbins's *Diet for a New America: How Your Food Choices Affect Your Health, Your Happiness and the Future of Life on Earth* offer real hope to individuals willing to commit to their health and to their lives.

Former President Bill Clinton is a stellar example of what an individual can accomplish by making a real commitment to change. After undergoing coronary artery bypass surgery and subsequent coronary stenting, Clinton adopted a plant-based, fat-free program that had been shown to reverse or at minimum to stay the ravages of coronary artery disease. His health has since improved dramatically. With Clinton, as with many others who make a serious commitment to their health, the results speak for themselves.

Cerebrovascular Disease

Cerebrovascular disease refers to brain dysfunction, which is related to diseases of the blood vessels supplying the brain. Hypertension and hypercholesterolemia are the two major pathologic contributors. Other risk factors for stroke include obesity, poor circulation, atrial fibrillation (irregular heartbeat), diabetes, age, smoking, excessive alcohol consumption, and recreational drug use.

Cerebrovascular diseases include transient ischemic attacks (TIA) or temporary diminution of blood supply to the brain and a stroke or permanent loss of blood flow to an area of the brain leading to sustained neurological damage. This permanent damage can be due either to loss of blood flow (ischemic stroke) or to bleeding within the brain (hemorrhagic stroke).

According to the World Health Organization, more than five million people die of stroke worldwide each year. This is a scary statistic, especially considering that many of the risk factors that could lead to stroke include unhealthy lifestyle choices. There are many warning signs of a stroke, and it is important to recognize these signs, so you can seek treatment immediately.

The following are the major warning signs of stroke:

- A loss of feeling in the face, arms, or legs. This could also manifest as a sudden weakness in these areas.

- Slurred or incoherent speech, drooling, or trouble comprehending simple instructions.

- Difficulty with motor skills, sudden dizziness, or a loss of equilibrium.

- Vision problems in one eye or both eyes.

- An intense and sudden headache with no logical cause.

Peripheral Vascular Disease

Peripheral vascular disease (PVD) refers to disease of the large arteries that supply the extremities of the body. It can result from atherosclerosis (plaque accumulation) or inflammation of the blood vessel walls leading to stenosis (narrowing of the blood vessel), embolism (movement of a blood clot or fat globule), or thrombosis (blood clot formation). The end result is the occlusion of a distal blood vessel leading to diminished blood flow to the limb, resulting in claudication (pain either with activity or at rest) and eventually necrosis or gangrene.

Risk factors contributing to peripheral vascular disease are the same as the ones for coronary artery disease and cerebrovascular disease. Hypertension, hypercholesterolemia, diabetes, and smoking head the list. Other risk factors are age, male gender, obesity, prior heart attacks or strokes, family history of atherosclerotic disease, and increased markers of inflammation. The prevalence of PVD in the general population is 12 to 14 percent, but this percentage increases to over 20 percent in those over the age of seventy.

MECHANICAL FUNCTION: THE PUMP

The second broad category of cardiac dysfunction involves malfunction of the pump, or the muscular function of the heart. Dysfunction of the heart muscle leads broadly to the development of congestive heart failure. There are two components of pump function: one involving contraction of the heart, and the second involving relaxation of the heart. Dysfunction that involves the contraction ability of the heart is known as systolic heart failure, whereas dysfunction involving the relaxation of the heart is known as diastolic heart failure.

Congestive Heart Failure

Congestive heart failure (CHF) is the condition in which the heart fails to adequately pump blood to the tissues of the body, leading to the deprivation of oxygen to the organs and to the accumulation of fluid within the tissues, particularly the lungs, liver, and lower extremities. CHF can be caused either by the heart being too weak to pump enough blood to the body's blood and tissues (a condition known as systolic dysfunction) or by the stiffening of the heart's ventricles (called diastolic dysfunction).

Common causes of CHF are coronary artery disease, cardiomyopathy (the weakening of the heart muscle), high blood pressure, valvular disease, congenital heart disease, and the overconsumption of alcohol and other toxins. Symptoms include shortness of breath, swelling of the abdomen or lower extremities, coughing, fatigue, dizziness, and sudden death.

Nearly five million Americans live with congestive heart failure, and an additional 500,000 cases are diagnosed each year. It is the leading cause of hospitalization in patients over the age of sixty-five. Heart failure has a bleak prognosis: nearly half of the people diagnosed with it die within five years. The disease accounts for approximately 287,000 deaths annually, with sudden death being a common occurrence among those cases.

ELECTRICAL CIRCUITRY SYSTEM

The third broad category of dysfunction involves the electrical circuitry of the heart. This could be likened to the electrical wiring necessary for certain types of machinery to function. It is the pathway through which our nervous system both commands the heart muscle to contract and dictates the speed of those contractions, or the heart rate. Without this pathway to transport the signals, the heart muscle would not turn on.

The electrical circuitry system starts with the sinoatrial (SA) node. I like to refer to this node as the commander in chief of the electrical system.

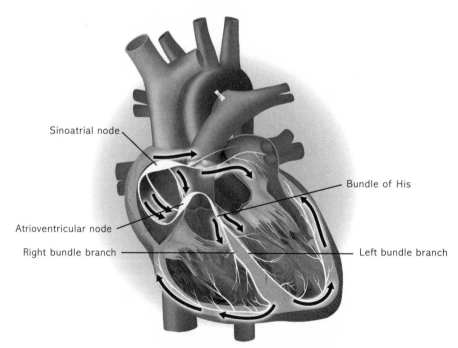

Sinoatrial node

Bundle of His

Atrioventricular node

Right bundle branch

Left bundle branch

Fig. 2-1   The Heart's Electrical Circuitry System

The SA node sends an impulse to the atrioventricular (AV) node, which functions like the lieutenant general of the system. From there, the impulse is further relayed down a right and a left bundle branch to the cardiac cells, which are the soldiers of the system.

Earlier, I explained how the cells of the heart work together in a coordinated fashion, much in the same way that a regiment of soldiers might march together as a coordinated unit. When a group of those soldiers or cells falls out of line or stops listening to the SA node, different forms of arrhythmias can occur.

Arrhythmias take the form of isolated or skipped heartbeats, and they can originate in either the top chamber or the bottom chamber of the heart. Many forms of arrhythmia are not dangerous.

Among its serious forms, the most common type is atrial fibrillation, which involves the rapid conduction and contractility of the top chambers of the heart (the atria), leading to chaotic, irregular rhythm in the bottom chambers of the heart (the ventricles). Other dangerous forms of arrhythmias include ventricular tachycardia and ventricular fibrillation, which are both fast rhythm arrhythmias (tachyarrhythmia). Slow rhythm arrhythmias (bradyarrhythmia) include sinus node dysfunction and second- and third-degree heart block.

HYPERTENSION: THE SILENT KILLER

AN EXECUTIVE EXPERIENCE

For years, Stephen ignored his high blood pressure. It had been almost a decade since he was first informed of the diagnosis. Initially he had been started on medication, but the treatment left him feeling fatigued.

Stephen was a high-level executive and worked extremely long, arduous hours. He could not be bothered with controlling his blood pressure, especially when he felt great and had no complaints. He exercised several days a week, was physically fit, and only had ten extra pounds of weight. He ate fairly well, or so he thought. He was mistrusting of the measurements he received in the doctor's office, and he always had an excuse for the elevated readings: just rushed here from work, on a tight deadline, the doctor's office makes me nervous.

Despite his doctor's urging, Stephen eventually stopped taking his medications and attending his routine physicals altogether. One morning, he awoke with a terrible headache and soon found himself vomiting. Something was clearly amiss. His wife called 911, but by the time they reached the emergency room, Stephen's speech was already impaired.

I met Stephen and his wife two weeks later. Stephen still had impaired speech. He had difficulty concentrating, couldn't form clear sentences, and had both short- and long-term memory loss. In addition, he was discharged from the hospital with the diagnosis of both heart failure and renal failure.

Six months later, Stephen was still on disability and attending rehab. He was increasingly frustrated and occasionally outright hostile and angry about his situation.

What happened to Stephen was a result of hypertension, the term we use for abnormally high blood pressure. It is called the "silent killer" because it does not develop overnight. Rather, it creeps up over a long period of time and is often clinically "silent," meaning that it does not have any warning symptoms.

Data collected by the CDC's Division of Heart Disease and Stroke Prevention in 2010 suggests that the prevalence of high blood pressure among adults, children, and teens is increasing. Recent statistics show that 77.6 percent of those with hypertension are aware that they have it, 67.9 percent of them are doing something to treat it, and 44.1 percent have achieved blood pressure control.

"Although hypertension is relatively easy to prevent, simple to diagnose, and relatively inexpensive to treat, it remains the second leading cause of death among Americans, and as such should rightly be called a neglected disease," noted Dr. David W. Fleming, the director and health officer for public health at Seattle and King County.

Hypertension is a tricky diagnosis because it isn't a static number. Your blood pressure fluctuates throughout the day. To compensate for that, I have a forty-point rule where I ask my patients to take their resting blood pressure and add forty points to that number. If you can comfortably add forty points and still have reasonable blood pressure, then the likelihood of significant hypertension is low.

The most common structural abnormality associated with hypertension is a thick heart muscle. When exposed to a high workload or burden, the heart will start to show structural changes.

Think of the heart muscle as you would think about your bicep. Your heart contracts approximately one hundred thousand times daily. That is equivalent to doing one hundred thousand curls nonstop, twenty-four hours a day, seven days a week, 365 days a year. Would your biceps rather lift five pounds of weight or fifty pounds of weight? If it is fifty pounds of weight, just how long do you think the muscle can sustain that load before giving up or tiring out?

That is in essence what happens to cause heart failure in hypertensive heart disease. The heart starts to give up and pump out less blood. That does not mean that the underlying heart muscle is weak. Rather, it is a sign that the heart is straining under a heavy workload. If you release the workload, the strength is usually still intact. I can always tell whether a person has high blood pressure just by looking at the thickness of the heart muscle—the same way that you can tell that a body builder lifts weights, even if you do not see him or her working out.

Hypertension is a major risk factor for cardiovascular disease. It also has a high association with other risk factors such as hypercholesterolemia, diabetes, insulin resistance, and impaired glucose metabolism.

According to the Joint National Committee on Prevention, Detection, Evaluation, and Treatment of High Blood Pressure, treating high blood pressure aggressively can prevent cardiovascular disease. Even though hypertension is easy to diagnose, the statistics show that adequate blood pressure control is still woefully lacking. The reason is that many patients prefer simply living with high blood pressure instead of aggressively treating it.

Lowering your blood pressure isn't a pleasant experience. When your blood pressure drops to below what you're used to, you feel lethargic and fatigued while your body is adjusting to the new level. It's a bit like going from a high-pressure showerhead to one that barely drips. In the beginning, you feel like you're being cheated of energy. While these are not welcome symptoms, they are the necessary steps required to get the brain readjusted and have the set point recalibrated.

The fact is that if you have high blood pressure, you're going to have to pay the piper somewhere down the line. Either you can pay him now and tolerate the unease and occasional dizziness and fatigue as you acclimate to the lower blood pressure, or you can pay him later as early dementia, early memory lapse, renal failure, cardiac failure, and other detrimental structural changes to the body start to occur.

Part of the goal of hypertension prevention is recognizing its potential causes. Genetic factors, increased sodium intake, impaired vascular tone, lack of proper nutrients, thyroid or adrenal issues, inadequate sleep, alcohol intake, and stress levels are all contributors. But consideration should also be given to herbal supplements and any medications you might be taking (antidepressants, birth control pills, and hormone replacement, for example).

You can take a few approaches to reduce hypertension, and most of them have to do with healthy lifestyle modifications. Reduce any excess weight you may be carrying. Increase your intake of fruits, vegetables, and whole grains. Avoid fats. Reduce your calorie intake by cutting back on things like sugar, sugary beverages, refined starches, saturated fats, and trans fats. Also reduce your sodium intake to meet dietary guidelines, increase your consumption of potassium-rich fruits and vegetables, and increase your physical activity. Aggressive drug therapy is another approach recommended by the Institute of Medicine, in combination with lifestyle changes.

Beyond these standard dietary recommendations, the American Heart Association (AHA) Professional Education Committee of the Council for High Blood Pressure Research, the Council on Cardiovascular and Stroke Nursing, the Council on Epidemiology and Prevention, and the Council on Nutrition, Physical Activity and Metabolism in April 2013 addressed other non-pharmacological treatments that could have the potential to lower blood pressure.

The three broad categories analyzed were behavioral therapy, noninvasive procedures or devices, and exercise-based regimens. Reviewing the current available scientific evidence, the committee concluded that participating in moderate to high dynamic aerobic exercise for thirty minutes a day, five days a week should be recommended. They also deemed that device-guided breathing and dynamic resistance training, such as weight lifting and circuit training, were reasonable to recommend.

Finally, the council concluded that isometric handgrip exercises, transcendental meditation, and biofeedback techniques might likewise be considered for recommendation, whereas other meditation and relaxation techniques such as yoga and acupuncture did not carry evidence for being beneficial. Only one device to help achieve slow breathing has been approved by the FDA for over-the-counter distribution (www.resperate.com).

TYPE 2 DIABETES

A REMARKABLE RECOVERY

Randy, a forty-five-year-old patient, was at least one hundred pounds over his ideal body weight. He had been on insulin for more than twenty years. He worked in the film industry, which is marked by long, grueling hours and the infamous craft tables with a spread fit for kings. The many years of poor dietary habits, overfilled plates, an erratic eating schedule, long work hours, and a lack of exercise had taken their toll on him.

Randy was on multiple medications for blood pressure and cholesterol, and was looking to have two knee replacements. By the time he came to see me for shortness of breath, his own mortality and the effect of years of neglect and abuse were taking shape and providing him with great clarity.

When I told Randy that I had a diet program that was designed to address metabolic syndrome and insulin resistance, he was all ears. He was ready to make a significant commitment toward his health.

Over the next month as he texted me his daily blood sugar level, Randy made tremendous strides toward improving his health and modifying his diet. He learned an important lesson about how much influence his daily choices had on his blood sugar. Within one month, he was able to come off his insulin altogether, which was remarkable. When last I saw him, Randy was down seventy pounds from his initial starting weight.

Randy had been suffering from type 2 diabetes. Also known as noninsulin-dependent diabetes or adult-onset diabetes, type 2 diabetes is the most common form of the illness. It develops slowly over time. According to the AHA, type 2 diabetes was once found mainly in middle-aged people, but today an alarming number of cases are diagnosed in teenagers and young adults, as well.

Currently, diabetes affects close to thirty million of the United States population, and it is estimated that an additional seventy-nine million American adults aged twenty and older have pre-diabetes. Worldwide, diabetes is the fastest-spreading disease, with the incidence doubling in the past two decades. This has led the World Health Organization to declare diabetes a global epidemic.

Type 2 diabetes is directly linked to poor dietary habits, obesity, and inactivity, and if this condition is not identified and managed, it can be life threatening. If untreated, type 2 diabetes can lead to health conditions such as heart disease, stroke, kidney disease, liver disease, nerve damage, and blindness.

Diabetes accelerates the aging process and is associated with depression, a higher rate of Alzheimer's disease, and more cardiovascular diseases than are seen in the general public. The AHA reports that people with diabetes are two to four times more likely to have a heart attack or a stroke than people who do not have diabetes. In addition, 65 percent of people with diabetes die from these afflictions, making heart disease and stroke the leading causes of death for people who suffer from diabetes.

Type 2 diabetes is a condition where the body does not produce enough insulin, or where the body cannot use the insulin that it produces in an efficient way. When you consume sugar or glucose from food, your body uses insulin, which is produced in the pancreas, to transport the glucose to cells in the body. Those cells then store that glucose and use it as a source of energy. If your pancreas does not produce enough insulin, or if the cells in your liver, fat, or muscles do not respond properly to the insulin (a condition called insulin resistance), then glucose builds up in the bloodstream.

Too much glucose in the bloodstream causes a condition called hyperglycemia, which can thicken the blood vessels and make it difficult for blood and oxygen to flow to the heart and brain. This can result in heart attacks and strokes. People with type 2 diabetes are also at a much higher risk of obesity, high blood pressure, high levels of bad LDL (low-density lipoprotein) cholesterol and triglycerides, and low levels of good HDL (high-density lipoprotein) cholesterol.

Because type 2 diabetes can be so dangerous when it is not properly managed, it is important to recognize the warning signs of this disease. The following are some common symptoms of diabetes:

- Constant hunger and thirst

- Frequent urination

- Unexplained fatigue or exhaustion

- Blurry vision

- Pain, numbness, or tingling in the hands and/or feet

- Dry mouth

- Infections that heal slowly

- Irregular heart rate

- Erectile dysfunction

As in Randy's case, the main causes of type 2 diabetes are excessive body weight or obesity, lack of exercise, and poor diet. The more weight you are carrying, the harder it is for your body to use insulin to carry glucose to the body's cells.

According to the Centers for Disease Control and Prevention, 95 percent of diabetes cases are caused by obesity and inactivity. Diabetes is also passed down genetically, so if someone in your family suffers from type 2 diabetes, the chances that you will develop this condition are high. Other risk factors for diabetes include race (type 2 diabetes is more prevalent in populations of black, Hispanic, or Asian-American people), age (the older you are, the higher your chances are of developing diabetes), pregnancy, lack of sleep, high blood pressure, and cardiovascular disease.

The good news is that type 2 diabetes is easily preventable. By following a healthy diet and exercising regularly, you can maintain a healthy weight and avoid diabetes. Even if you do develop diabetes, exercise and diet can play a huge part in alleviating the symptoms. If you are diagnosed with type 2 diabetes, it is important to monitor your blood sugar levels so that you can adapt your diet and exercise plan accordingly. There are many anti-diabetic medications that your doctor may prescribe to treat the symptoms. Insulin can also be injected into the body to regulate blood sugar levels.

However, no medication can cure or reverse diabetes, and medications often come with multiple side effects, including weight gain. The only treatment shown to be effective in changing the natural history or progression of the disease is to enact significant lifestyle changes, with exercise and dietary modification. Dr. Neal Barnard's *Program for Reversing Diabetes* and Dr. Joel Fuhrman's *The End of Diabetes* provide in-depth, non-drug-based methodologies for addressing diabetes.

Specific foods will help control dangerous spikes in blood sugar. Beans are high on this list. Whole-grain foods, non-starchy vegetables, wild salmon or sardines, egg whites, non-dairy yogurt, cinnamon, ginseng, ginkgo biloba, fenugreek seeds, bilberry leaves, salt bush, curry leaves, avocados, almonds, and healing drinks such as water, tea, and black coffee are all high on the list.

Alternative natural remedies, including acupuncture and yoga, can also help to manage diabetes. We will explore more natural remedies and dietary paths to health in later chapters.

Although type 2 diabetes can be treated, it is obviously better to prevent it altogether. The best thing you can do to avoid this health condition is to eat a healthy, nutritious diet and to exercise on a regular basis. Be aware of the symptoms of diabetes, and see a doctor if you suspect you may be pre-diabetic or diabetic.

HIGH CHOLESTEROL: THE STORY ABOUT FAT

Our bodies need cholesterol to perform basic functions. However, too much cholesterol can lead to serious health problems. The condition of having too much cholesterol in the body is called high cholesterol, and it can lead to problems such as atherosclerosis (hardening of the arteries), angina, heart attacks, and stroke.

Many people have high cholesterol, but are unaware that they may be at risk for cardiovascular disease. According to the CDC, one in six American adults has dangerously high levels of cholesterol, and these individuals have a 50 percent greater risk of developing heart disease than people with healthy cholesterol levels.

Cholesterol is a fatty, waxy substance produced by the liver and found in certain foods. It is circulated in the body through blood plasma, and it is found in all the cells in the body.

Our bodies can produce all the cholesterol that we need. However, certain foods provide additional cholesterol that can be used or stored in the body for energy. We need cholesterol for metabolic functions, such as producing hormones and bile; absorbing fat-soluble vitamins such as A, D, E, and K; converting sunshine into vitamin D; insulating the nerves; and protecting and maintaining the outer layer of cell membranes.

Triglycerides are also related to cholesterol. These are essentially fats that are consumed in the food you eat. If you eat more calories than your body needs for energy, your body will convert the extra calories from the foods into triglycerides. The triglycerides are then either broken down in the liver and transported throughout the body or stored in fat cells. If your body needs extra energy later, it can draw upon these fat stores for fuel. However, excessive caloric intake and inactivity can lead to an overproduction of bad LDL cholesterol, which can put you at risk of coronary heart disease.

People with high cholesterol have a much higher risk of developing coronary heart disease. Cholesterol within blood vessels acts like a Band-Aid over the damaged endothelium or lining of blood vessels. Therefore, damage to the blood-vessel lining from the sheer stress of hypertension or damage from high blood sugar and insulin levels will lead to more accumulation of cholesterol in the lining of the blood vessels. Over time, this bad LDL cholesterol builds up in the arteries, forming plaque that prevents the arteries from pumping blood and oxygen to the heart.

Plaque in the arterial walls can also cause blood clots to form, which can cut off blood to the brain and the heart. When the heart cannot receive the blood it needs, the muscle starts to die, which is what we call a heart attack. If the brain does not receive sufficient blood and oxygen, it also begins to die, which is known as a stroke. People with high cholesterol may also exhibit yellow patches of cholesterol deposits on the skin. However, many people show no symptoms whatsoever of high cholesterol, and only find out that they have it after it is too late.

Some of the main causes of high cholesterol include an unhealthy diet that is high in saturated fats, being overweight or obese, a lack of exercise, genetics, excessive alcohol intake, smoking, an underactive thyroid gland, kidney and liver disease, high blood pressure, and diabetes. Insulin resistance and high levels of insulin can also contribute to the problem, since insulin is the key that allows triglycerides to form in the first place.

Men are more susceptible to increased cholesterol levels, as are women who experience early menopause. That being said, people of all ages can have high cholesterol.

A recent CDC study revealed that one in ten youths between the ages of six and nineteen has elevated cholesterol levels in America. The American Pediatric Association recently updated its recommendation of when children should be assessed for elevated cholesterol, stating that all children with a family history of cardiovascular disease or hyperlipidemia should be screened beginning soon after the age of two and no later than the age of ten.

The good thing about high cholesterol is that it can easily be prevented. The best way to manage and maintain healthy cholesterol levels is by eating a nutritious diet of whole grains, fruits, vegetables, nuts, seeds, and low-fat proteins. Try to cut out saturated fats and unnecessary sugar and salt.

Some foods known to lower cholesterol include artichoke leaves, basil, ginger, and turmeric. A combination of honey and cinnamon has also been touted to affect cholesterol lowering, though it is important to note that the cinnamon used for this purpose should be true cinnamon—or Ceylon cinnamon—which has the medicinal effect. Plant sterols and dietary fiber also work to lower cholesterol in the body. Other ways to lower cholesterol include exercising regularly, losing weight, decreasing alcohol consumption, quitting smoking, and getting sufficient sleep.

Certain drugs can effectively lower cholesterol levels in the body. It is important to discuss medications with your doctor before taking any cholesterol-lowering drugs. I always tell my patients that medications do not treat high cholesterol, they only lower the measured laboratory numbers while on the medication. True treatment and even reversal comes when the person successfully changes his or her habits.

One example is a patient of mine named Tricia, who had significant triglyceridemia to the point that she was having recurring bouts of pancreatitis. Even with multiple potent medications, we were only able to successfully lower her triglyceride levels to 500 milligrams per deciliter (normal is under 150 mg/dl). Tricia had always been counseled to modify her diet, but had been having a difficult time complying with any regimen.

She enrolled in our weight-loss management program, and within two months, even before achieving significant weight loss, she had appreciably modified her triglycerides, which were lower than they had been in decades. Tricia learned that as potent as drugs are, the real power to enact true change lies within us.

METABOLIC SYNDROME

Metabolic syndrome is a condition that affects more than forty-seven million adults in America, and that number is rapidly rising according to the National Heart, Lung, and Blood Institute, a division of the National Institutes of Health.

Metabolic syndrome is thought to be the leading contributor to the development of heart attacks and strokes, as its diagnosis consolidates the presence of the major risk factors for the development of atherosclerosis, namely obesity, hypertension, diabetes, and dyslipidemia. A Swedish study revealed that men over fifty who had metabolic syndrome were 60 percent more likely to suffer heart failure than those without this condition.

People who are diagnosed with metabolic syndrome suffer from at least three out of five of the following health conditions:

- Excess fat, particularly around the waist, and a high Body Mass Index (BMI). If your BMI is more than 25, you are considered overweight. A BMI of more than 30 indicates obesity.

- High blood pressure. You should aim to have a blood pressure reading of below 130 over 85.

- High levels of triglycerides. For optimum health, your triglyceride levels should be below 150.

- Low levels of high-density lipoprotein (HDL) cholesterol. Your HDL levels should be above 40 for men and above 50 for women.

- High blood glucose levels or insulin resistance. Healthy blood glucose levels are below 100.

The main causes of metabolic syndrome are lifestyle choices. These include an unhealthy diet, excess fat intake, and inactivity. In addition, genetics and age play a role. The basic pathophysiology is insulin resistance, and research shows that stress is a contributing factor. According to the AHA, one in three Americans has metabolic syndrome, and these people are twice as likely to have a heart attack or stroke and five times as likely to develop diabetes as people who do not suffer from this condition.

The good news is that metabolic syndrome is preventable and can even be reversed if it is diagnosed in time. The best thing you can do to avoid this condition is lead a healthy life. This means eating a nutritious diet of fruits, vegetables, whole grains, nuts, and seeds, and cutting out fats whenever possible.

A comparison of a typical Western diet of refined grains, processed meats, fried foods, poor-quality red meat, and soda versus a Mediterranean diet of cruciferous vegetables such as broccoli and cabbage, carotenoid vegetables (carrots, pumpkins), fruit, fish, seafood, poultry, whole grains, and low-fat dairy showed an 18 percent higher risk of developing metabolic syndrome on the typical Western diet. Furthermore, there was a relative reduction of approximately 30 percent in heart attacks, strokes, and death among high-risk persons who were initially free of cardiovascular disease.

Exercise also goes a long way toward a healthy heart and can help shed those excess pounds around the waist. Studies of a Targeted Risk Reduction Intervention through Defined Exercise (STRRIDE) performed at Duke Medical Center suggest that getting at least thirty minutes of brisk walking in a day, six days a week, can lower the risk of metabolic syndrome by 50 percent. If lifestyle changes are not making a significant difference in reversing metabolic syndrome, then more aggressive intervention by way of medical attention may be necessary to reset the pendulum.

If you find yourself meeting with frustration with little gain from your lifestyle interventions, your physician should be able to more effectively guide you to a structured lifestyle and dietary intervention that will stay the progression of, and possibly even reverse, metabolic syndrome.

THE OBESITY EPIDEMIC

Obesity is a very serious health problem that is rising in many countries around the world. A person is considered obese if he or she is 20 percent or more above his or her ideal body weight. The body mass index (BMI) is a good indicator of a healthy weight. If your BMI is 30 or higher, you are considered obese.

Excess weight takes its toll on the body in many ways, which is why obesity is directly linked to hypertension, high cholesterol, atherosclerosis, heart failure, stroke, diabetes, sleep apnea, certain types of cancer, osteoarthritis, fatty liver disease, insulin resistance, and gout. The only good thing about obesity is that it is preventable and can be treated.

The American Medical Association (AMA) in June 2013 declared obesity a chronic disease, "requiring a range of medical interventions to advance treatment and prevention." Up to this point, the AMA had considered obesity to be a major public health concern but had not defined it as a disease, thereby limiting insurance coverage to combat this serious health issue. Currently, obesity-related health-care expenses range in the billions of dollars each year.

Obesity is caused mainly by eating too many calories and not exercising. When you eat an excessive amount of calories, your body stores the fats and sugars within fat cells. If you do not use up these sources of energy through physical activity, you start to build fat around the waist and all over the body. In addition, a diet that is heavy in saturated fats, trans fats, and cholesterol can lead to weight gain.

While some people may be overweight or obese as a result of genetics or preexisting medical conditions such as an underactive thyroid gland, the main culprit of this disease is an unhealthy lifestyle.

I'd like to take a moment to introduce the concept of calorie density. Calorie density refers to the amount of calories that exist in a given weight of food. Ideally, you want to consume foods that are nutritionally dense, meaning that they contain the highest amount of vitamins, minerals, and phytonutrients while simultaneously containing the least amount of calories per ounce or pound of food (known as low calorie density). Foods that meet these criteria are usually high in water content and low in fat content, and they provide you with higher satisfaction in combination with a lower consumption of calories.

Non-starchy vegetables have the lowest calorie density, followed by fruits, starchy vegetables, intact whole grains, and legumes. Processed carbohydrates, sugars, nuts, and seeds have higher calorie densities, and oils have the greatest number of calories per ounce. A 2007 report from the American Cancer Institute and the World Cancer Research Fund recommended lowering the average calorie density to 567 calories per pound.

One of the major effects of obesity on health is an increased risk of heart attack and stroke. When you are obese, your heart needs to work harder to supply blood to the extra tissues and cells in the body. This puts a great deal of strain on your heart muscle.

In addition, too much fat in the body causes bad LDL cholesterol levels to soar, which leads to a buildup of plaque in the arteries. Atherosclerosis, or hardened arteries, makes it harder for the heart to pump blood to the rest of the body. This can eventually cause the heart muscle to die.

In addition, blood clots from blocked arteries can cut off the blood supply to the brain, causing a stroke. Studies show that obesity is also linked to heart failure.

The Framingham Heart Study followed nearly six thousand overweight and obese people for fourteen years, and looked at their rates of heart failure. Even after researchers corrected the study for other risk factors such as hypertension and previous cardiac episodes, they found that the overweight people had a 34 percent higher chance of experiencing heart failure than people who maintained a healthy weight. For the obese people, the chances of heart failure were a shocking 104 percent greater than the people who were at a healthy weight.

Obesity puts a strain on almost every system and cell in the body. For example, excess weight puts pressure on the bones and joints, eventually causing osteoarthritis. Many obese people are diagnosed with chronic obstructive pulmonary disease (COPD) or sleep apnea. When the arteries are clogged, blood and oxygen cannot circulate efficiently, making it difficult for the organs to function properly and for toxins to be flushed out of the body.

A buildup in toxins can lead to certain forms of cancer and can suppress the immune system. The fact that obesity affects the entire body all at once makes this a very serious health condition.

Obesity, which is becoming a worldwide epidemic, is 100 percent preventable. The best way to avoid gaining an excessive amount of weight is by eating a healthy diet and getting plenty of exercise.

Cutting out foods that are high in saturated fats and cholesterol, and eating a variety of fresh fruits and vegetables, whole grains, seeds, and nuts, should be the first step in staving off obesity. Experts recommend doing moderate exercise at least five days a week for thirty minutes at a time. Monitoring your caloric intake is another way to make sure that you are not consuming more food than your body can use for energy.

One of the common pitfalls when it comes to achieving weight loss is not paying attention to your body and how it responds to various fuel sources. While I don't subscribe to the premise of metabolic typing, which states that people have distinct metabolisms that are best served by different nutritional profiles (protein type, carbohydrates type, or mixed type), I do believe that each body has particular sensitivities and preferences for foods that should not be ignored.

Careful attention should be paid to how the body responds to different macronutrient food sources, particularly in the areas of energy, satiety, digestion, sleeping pattern, emotions, physical appearance, and food preference. It is important to determine which macronutrients work best for your body, as it becomes less likely that you will overeat when you are providing the proper nutrients to your body in the first place.

My patients have enjoyed tremendous success in addressing their obesity and metabolic syndrome challenges. Much of the credit for that goes to each individual's mindset and determination to be the person who creates the desired changes. Determining the right course of action requires clarity of vision as well as the elimination of limiting beliefs that will impede success.

Through this greater understanding of the big picture, I have created a truly exceptional program to help my clients with their weight-loss endeavors and their health goals. The method I use is the Ideal Protein protocol, which was developed more than twenty-five years ago by Dr. Tran Tien Chanh. It is an FDA-approved, highly calibrated protocol designed to enact metabolic changes within the body that then enable the patient to realize results for their efforts.

The Ideal Protein diet is a four-phase protocol that focuses on the goal of helping dieters stabilize their pancreas and blood sugar levels through a structured meal and lifestyle program.

The core principle of Ideal Protein is to learn to live off your body's own fat stores while maintaining muscle mass. Central to the protocol are the improvement of insulin sensitivity, the reversal of metabolic syndrome, the detoxification of the body, and the shifting of the body's pH balance toward alkaline food. Withdrawal of high glucose and insulin levels leads to a restoration of leptin sensitivity, therefore aiding in establishing satiety. The predictable fat burn releases a high amount of energy, and therefore the body does not go into a hibernation mode and slow down metabolism.

When I first learned of the Ideal Protein protocol, I tried it myself. I noticed that my body metabolism increased, improving my body's rate of digesting food. In two months, I shed twenty pounds, which have continued to stay off, despite a heavy work schedule. As a family, we also started eating more raw and whole foods, which has increased our energy levels.

When I started to truly appreciate all the positive changes that I had made in myself as well as in my patients, I incorporated a more holistic approach into my cardiology practice, steering my patients to find a way to live better and get healthier.

Our approach is multifaceted, providing nutritional counseling that includes educating our patients on plant-based nutrition, providing Dr. Sears's L.E.A.N. and Prime-Time Health workshops, administering the Ideal Protein protocol, and offering life-mastery coaching to clear limiting beliefs and establish a vibrational match for the vision that our patients are trying to achieve.

More than a year after establishing this holistic approach into my practice, I founded Revitalize-U, our health and wellness center. Having the program at my office for patients who were interested in taking positive steps to improve their overall health and well-being has allowed me to guide many successful clients to titrate down or come off blood pressure, cholesterol, and diabetes medications.

The program has truly been a blessing and has provided me with much professional and personal satisfaction. In the first two years alone, our enrolled clientele of more than four hundred patients achieved a combined weight-loss total of over ten thousand pounds!

Achieving and maintaining a healthy BMI may be difficult, but it can add years to your life and improve your image and self-confidence.

THE LIE ABOUT SMOKING

A patient of mine, Tom, told me a story once. He and his older brother had been chain-smokers since they were thirteen, going through as many as three packs of cigarettes a day. One of them had emphysema, and the other had lung cancer.

Tom's older brother met a younger woman and had a child, at which point he just quit smoking cold turkey. About seven years after he quit, he was visiting Tom and, while they were out on the porch, had ten cigarettes—just for old times' sake. That same night in his hotel gymnasium while he was working out, Tom's brother dropped dead of a massive heart attack.

So how do you smoke three packs of cigarettes a day for some fifty years, have emphysema without having heart disease, quit for seven years, and then after a ten-cigarette binge one night have a massive heart attack and die? That is how smoking works. It is idiosyncratic. It is a random risk, and you never know when the trigger will be pulled on the Russian roulette you are playing with your life.

According to the AHA, cigarette smoking is the most prolific preventable cause of premature death in the United States, accounting for 440,000 of the country's more than 2.4 million annual deaths. Smoking causes a buildup of fatty substances (called atheromas) in the arteries. Smoking and the carcinogens that come from it can lead to heart failure. Smoking also increases the risk of stroke.

I want to emphasize that the heart-attack risk associated with cigarette smoking is entirely random. It is like playing Las Vegas odds. It is different from lung cancer, where there is a dose-response risk. If you smoke three packs per day, then you have a much, much higher risk of getting lung cancer than the person who picks up an occasional cigarette.

However, with smoking and heart attacks, one puff of one cigarette can cause a heart attack if it is your unlucky day. As in the case of Tom's brother, the fact that you have gotten away with smoking for thirty years does not guarantee that your next cigarette will not cause a heart attack.

Most people who smoke are well aware of their risk. That is not the motivator that they need to quit. I often find that patients want to quit or at least try to quit smoking, but they do not know how to go about it, or they fear failure.

My job is to give them a sense of empowerment. My words are meant to be motivational and educational. I never imply that stopping smoking is easy, because it is not. I acknowledge that it is a very, very difficult process.

What I impress on my patients more than anything else is this: smoking is not addictive. That is the big lie about smoking. Patients as well as physicians have this notion that there are chemical pathways and brain pathways that make you feel compelled to smoke. Therefore, physicians offer alternatives such as the patch, gum, Nicorette, Chantix, or other pharmacological means to break out of the smoking cycle. I feel that taking this type of approach is detrimental because it feeds into the notion that the patient does not have absolute control over the decision to smoke or not.

The reality is that individuals do have control over this decision. Addiction is defined by biochemical dependency: the body is dependent on the substance for which there is an addiction. Dependency is defined by withdrawal symptoms at the absence of that dependency. So for example, alcohol is addictive for some people: they get tremors, shakes, or even seizures when alcohol is withdrawn from them.

> To stop any habit, you need an equally powerful motivator. In life, there are two things that move us to action: pleasure and the avoidance of pain.

Caffeine can be addictive, too: all those who are addicted to this drug are at risk for predictable, uniform caffeine-withdrawal headaches. Cocaine, heroin, and speed are also addictive substances. To combat them, we provide a synthetic substance known as methadone to drug addicts to prevent them from suffering from seizures, strokes, or even death as they detox from an addictive substance. In all of these cases, the withdrawal symptoms are defined by a predictable biochemical response.

By contrast, there is no such uniform response to nicotine withdrawal. Some people stop completely without any problem at all. Others hallucinate. Still others develop hostile reactions to things, or they overeat. There is absolutely no consistency in the supposed withdrawal symptoms of nicotine.

So do you want to know what I call all these reactions? I call them adult temper tantrums. You are raging against yourself, trying to manipulate yourself, doing that negative self-talk to defeat yourself and to get yourself to give in. In the end, you are your worst enemy.

I tell my patients that the actual act of quitting smoking is easy, once you are clear about your decision. With clarity and definiteness of purpose, there is no need to throw

> Will is the ability of our mind to command our body to do anything we ask of it.

tantrums or to manipulate and fight yourself. If the tantrums do occur, the best way to deal with them is not to feed into them.

Even young children know that if a parent is weak they are going to bang their heads, rage, scream, cry, and do whatever it takes to get the result they want. However, when the parent is firm, then all of sudden that tantrum is over. They go off and play, and they forget about the thing they were raging about. If children can understand that there is no point in throwing a tantrum if they are not going to get what they want, then an adult can be smart enough to do the same.

Many will disagree with my analysis, arguing that nicotine acts as a stimulant within the brain, accounting for its addictive properties. My response is that there are many things in life that give us pleasure and that turn on endorphins that cause biochemical changes and signals within the brain, but we don't call all pleasure addictions. If we did, we would suddenly find that we have addictions to food, sex, porn, money, electronic games, sucking our thumbs, or holding our favorite teddy bear.

True addictions that cause biochemical dependency should have predictable, reproducible, definable, and uniform withdrawal symptoms in the absence of that dependency. We may choose to view porn in the middle of the night in the basement, but we aren't going to do it in the middle of the afternoon at the office, in full view of our coworkers and our boss. That is a fully conscious choice, and I would not classify that as an addiction. It is a habit.

To stop any habit, you need an equally powerful motivator. In life, there are two things that move us to action: pleasure and the avoidance of pain. The avoidance of pain is the more potent stimulator. Many patients who have tried unsuccessfully many times to quit smoking do so successfully the day they have their first heart attack, stroke, or bypass surgery, or are informed that they have lung cancer. All of a sudden, the "addiction" no longer exists, because they now have definiteness of purpose and clarity of vision.

I always ask my patients if they are ready to make a commitment. If they are not, that is okay. They need to be ready. I ask them to be honest with themselves, which is even more important than being honest with me. I tell them to not play the game of starting and stopping, quitting multiple times for a short duration on every go-round.

If you are not ready, if you are going to struggle, then don't even fight with yourself, and don't live in guilt. Just work toward preparing yourself mentally for the day that you will quit. If my patients do decide to commit, I always ask them to shake my hand on that, as it adds a symbolic significance to the commitment.

Again, commitment speaks to the power of the mind. Henry Ford said it best: "If you think you can do a thing or if you think you can't do a thing, you are right."

It's not about willpower, which implies force. It's about will. Will is the ability of our mind to command our body to do anything we ask of it. When we are mentally ready, we can command ourselves using free will to do anything we desire, including the cessation of smoking. Success comes from knowing that what we are undertaking is being done out of free will.

CHAIN-SMOKER'S EPIPHANY

I met Joseph, aged forty, when he came in for an evaluation. His father had died of a heart attack at the age of forty. Joseph had two boys and was a chain-smoker.

I had my usual discussion with him regarding all the detrimental issues related to smoking, and I explained to him that smoking is not addictive. He was not ready to absorb that information. It happened that our treadmill was broken that day, so we scheduled him to come back in two weeks.

On his return, there was this huge grin on his face, and I said, "You quit."

He replied, "Yeah. You know doctor, I went home and did not really think about our discussion. I really had no interest in stopping smoking." That night, after he'd had his dinner with his wife and boys and they were all sitting down in the living room playing Nintendo, his wife suddenly became hysterical.

"What did the doctor say?" she asked him.

Joseph said, "Nothing. I am going back in two weeks for the stress test."

Then it dawned on him why his wife was hysterical. For the nineteen years that he and his wife had known each other, he had never gone through a meal without going out to the porch afterward and having his cigarettes. She had never seen him make it through funerals, weddings, or even the births of their children without going out to have his puffs.

So the fact that he'd skipped the cigarettes that night and gone straight to sitting down with his boys after dinner was like some kind of death sentence to her. She thought that the doctor had given him some horrific news, and that that had to be why he was not smoking. After all, his father had died when he was forty. "She asked me why I wasn't smoking," Joseph reported. "I just said, 'I don't need to.'"

I tell his story because he truly had an epiphany that night. In that moment of pure honesty where he said "I don't need to," he realized that he did not need to smoke not just that night, but also yesterday, or the day before that, or the day after that. Seeing his wife and his two children and realizing that he himself had grown up at that age without a father, he made the decision in that moment that he did not need to smoke. "Doc, it was as simple and as easy as you told me it would be. I did not think about it, I did not give it a second thought. I just said I did not need to, and I stopped."

In reality, the beauty of the heart is that it has cadence and rhythm, and that it acts like a melodious symphony echoing our physical, emotional, and mental state.

That is why I tell people: do not fight yourself, do not struggle. If you are not ready, then you are not ready. In that moment of clarity when you make that decision, it will truly be as easy as that. The difficulty is in the decision itself. Once we make it, the rest is simple. We simply exercise our will.

BE STILL MY HEART

One last common heart condition that I want to discuss is arrhythmia. Arrhythmia is simply defined as a change in rhythm. Some arrhythmias are benign, and others fall into the malignant or serious category. You cannot always tell based on symptoms.

So, when I evaluate someone who is having palpitations, I segregate them into two broad categories: those who have a structurally normal heart and those who have a structurally abnormal heart due to coronary artery disease, hypertensive heart disease, valvular disease, cardiomyopathy, or congenital heart disease. The majority of patients I evaluate on a daily basis have a structurally normal heart.

If the heart structurally looks normal and there is no history suggesting prior events or pathology, then most of the time the palpitations are a result of things exterior to the heart, such as stress, anxiety, lack of sleep, caffeine, nicotine, alcohol, pain, euphoria, anemia—the list goes on and on and on.

Sometimes, however, none of these factors are present, and the palpitations occur randomly for no obvious reason other than perhaps that the stars and the moon are aligned or that the waves are in high tide. These random factors drive the heart to act up transiently.

Although palpitations are often an experience of a normally functioning heart, emotions, concerns, and fears can magnify the symptoms. They do this in a number of ways. Your emotions can cause a negative feedback loop, which can in turn cause adrenaline, cortisol, and other neurohormones and neurotransmitters to surge, leading to a physiologic internal stimulation of the heart. Your emotions also affect neurotransmitters within the brain, altering your level of perception and making you more aware of symptoms that otherwise might have been overlooked.

Oftentimes, when palpitations are only perceived during the evening and nighttime, that is a perception issue. The slight irregularity or skip is present throughout the day as well, but it goes unnoticed by the individual when he or she is active and distracted by the occurrences of the day.

Most people assume that the heart should act like a mechanical robot or a cuckoo clock: tick-tock, tick-tock, right on key. In reality, the beauty of the heart is that it has cadence and rhythm, and that it acts like a melodious symphony echoing our physical, emotional, and mental state. The heart can be quiet and imperceptible, or it can be pounding out of your chest.

When we are excited because our horse just won the Kentucky Derby or when we are having terrific sex, we think nothing of the pounding heart. However, if it is pounding at a time when we are quiet and supposedly not excited or anxious, then we assume that there is some pathology involved.

The heart can slow down when we are sad or depressed, or when we are sleeping, and it speeds up with stimulation, whether physical, mental, emotional, or stimulant driven.

A PATHOLOGICAL FEAR

Mary arrived in my office one day in tears. She had been sent over from the local urgent care center.

In the preceding month, she had had three emergency room visits, with her husband and two small children (ages two and four) in tow. She had been experiencing frightening palpitations, as if her heart were going to leap out of her chest. The symptoms occurred mostly at nighttime, occasionally shaking her from sleep. She feared leaving her two small children behind if something dreadful were to happen to her.

When I questioned her further, I discovered that she was nearing the anniversary of a harrowing illness that had taken place the year before, in which she had almost lost her life. Her cardiac evaluation was completely normal, but she could not be reassured. She was unwilling to consider that stress and the pathologic fear of mortality could be the driving forces of her symptoms.

She eventually needed to be placed on anxiolytic medication, and she put herself in the care of a therapist.

Fortunately, in the majority of the palpitation cases that I manage, the patients are reassured once I inform them that the arrhythmia they are experiencing is benign.

STUDENT'S COMFORT LEVEL

Sarah was a graduate nursing student in her final week of examinations. Over the preceding two months, she had been experiencing intermittent fluttering in her heart. It appeared to be random and not correlated with stress.

Sarah felt as though she were on top of her game and did not feel excessively stressed or overwhelmed by her workload. Since visiting her primary care physician and getting the referral to me, she had already started to feel an ease in her symptoms. Her electrocardiogram came back completely normal, and she had a structurally normal heart. I did not think a holter monitor was warranted and proceeded to reassure her of this.

She was accepting of the diagnosis of stress-induced heart palpitations, and was willing to put "Pandora" back into her box. I saw her back for a six-month follow-up, and she was pleased to report that she had passed all of her finals, and that the palpitations had pretty much resolved themselves as I had predicted they would.

I like to think of the heart as a very sensitive mood ring. In some ways, the heart is almost more sensitive than even our minds or our physical brains.

Consequently, at times people will say that they are not anxious, but their hearts suggest otherwise. Your heart senses something that you may not on a conscious level be aware of or be willing to admit to, and in reality there may be some underlying stress or anxiety going on there. It might even be the low-level anxiety over not knowing why you are feeling what you are feeling that drives the symptoms further.

Remember that we think with our conscious mind, but that our emotions are the gateway to our subconscious world. So when people come to see me for palpitations, the majority of the time, their symptoms are a reflection of some internal turmoil that they are going through, even though they might not even be aware of it on the conscious plane.

Healthy habits, such as eating the right foods, drinking plenty of water, exercising, and getting plenty of sleep, are a good way to deal with arrhythmia. Nine times out of ten, just knowing that you have a structurally normal heart, detoxifying your body, and incorporating healthy habits take care of the issue.

We do not need to know or understand why the palpitations or arrhythmia first started. We just need to know that it is no longer an issue. Sometimes the arrhythmia calms down and goes away out of the blue for no obvious reason just as quickly as it came. That is the beauty of nature.

My husband and I went to Germany for our honeymoon. I was in my mid-thirties, just finishing postgraduate medical training, and as such I had no time for luxury or pleasure spending. In Germany, however, we splurged and bought a $2,000 cuckoo clock. I was not used to spending even $200 on dispensable pleasure items, much less $2,000 on a clock!

MIND-BODY AXIS

VISUALIZE YOUR HEALTH

It is always easier for people to deal with the symptoms or ailments of the physical body than to deal with the deep-rooted emotions of their mental or spiritual body. It is far easier to come in complaining of palpitations. It is far easier to come in complaining of palpitations. Some people find it hard even to talk with their spouse, much less to the doctor, or even to acknowledge to themselves that they may be dealing with stress or emotional issues, which is driving their symptoms. Your body and your symptoms are physical manifestations of your entire being and reflect whether your mind, your emotions, your spirit, and your soul are in harmony. The body is talking to you. We just have to wake up and listen—not to mention learn the language so that we don't misinterpret the message.

> Once we recognize and conquer those limiting beliefs, the universe will deliver the right people and the right opportunities to allow the manifestation of the vision that we have stated with crystal-clear determination.

We came back home to our one-bedroom apartment, and all I ever heard was tick-tock, tick-tock, tick-tock, cuckoo, cuckoo, all night long. I used to lay there awake at two o'clock in the morning . . . three o'clock in the morning. For days and weeks I could not sleep. I would get up in the morning and shut it off, and my husband would click it back on again, saying that we had spent $2,000 on this lovely cuckoo clock and we had better darn well enjoy it.

It took a while, but once I finally managed to accept that this chirping bird was going to be a part of my life from now on, I just stopped hearing it. It became a natural part of my existence.

The same lesson holds true for arrhythmia. Certain things happen in our lives and in our bodies where all of a sudden, symptoms become manifested and start to be noticeable. If we pay attention to them, they take on a life of their own, and then all of a sudden what was relatively "out there" (external stimuli) becomes "in here" (internal stress).

Sometimes it is just a matter of accepting it as a part of your existence and not really worrying about it. Your refusal to focus on it can sometimes make the symptoms literally go away, simply because you no longer perceive them as abnormal. They become a part of normalcy.

The majority of the cases of symptomatic palpitations is benign and is otherwise known as sinus arrhythmia. A few others, however, can be serious. These serious forms of arrhythmia tend to occur later in age. The most common of them include atrial fibrillation, ventricular tachycardia, and ventricular fibrillation. In cases such as these, a pacemaker or defibrillator might be considered. Your medical professional can recommend a form of treatment that is appropriate to your situation.

THE BIG PICTURE

Emotional negativity can be a factor in many heart-related diseases. It's not the only thing to keep an eye on. Identifying and managing your risk factors are also paramount to maintaining heart health. A well-balanced combination of these mental and physical elements is your best bet to keeping your heart in tip-top shape.

Part of my work involves helping our clients get crystal clear as to the reason for their endeavors. Weight loss is a good example. It is not enough to say "I want to lose weight" or "I want to get healthier." Those goals are too vague. Specific goals are statements like, "I want to lose fifty pounds so I can come off my blood pressure and diabetes medications," "I want to fit into a size-six dress for my twenty-fifth high school reunion," or, "I want to go hiking and play soccer with my grandchildren."

By being clear and specific, you are invoking the Law of Attraction and the Law of Vibration by telling the universe in detail what you want and why. It is important to explore

MIND-BODY AXIS

HONE YOUR AWARENESS

One of the most important life-mastery skills is to notice what you are paying attention to or getting interested in. That which we pay attention to tells the universe our intention. So if your intention is not to experience palpitations, then don't fuel it by giving attention to it. Instead, choose to turn your attention toward something that you desire, and see what happens. Remember, we have 100 percent control over our thoughts, but oftentimes we do not exercise this awesome power to our advantage and instead use the power of the mind to torment ourselves or fill ourselves with fears, doubts, or physical symptoms. You can receive my free e-book 101 Positive Affirmations to Revitalize-U by visiting: www.drcynthia.com/affirmations.

any limiting beliefs you may hold, which may form the borders of our comfort zones and which can lead to anxiety, fear, or doubt when we start challenging those beliefs.

An easy way to identify limiting beliefs is to become an observer in the conversations that you have with others or with yourself and to notice anything that is negative. Ralph Waldo Emerson said, "Stand guard at the portal of your mind." It is so important to notice where we have placed our attention. If the predominant thought is that you have never successfully maintained weight loss, then the vibrational match for that thought or emotion will make that thought into a reality.

Once we recognize and conquer those limiting beliefs, the universe will deliver the right people and the right opportunities to allow the manifestation of the vision that we have stated with crystal-clear determination.

CHAPTER 3

FOOD FOR YOUR HEART

"Let your food be your medicine and let your medicine be your food."
—Hippocrates

A vital component of a healthy heart and longevity is a well-balanced diet. Most chronic diseases are primarily related to poor diets and lack of healthy lifestyles.

The benefits of a healthy diet are exceptional and revolve around looking better, feeling better, and living longer. In this chapter, you will learn how to eat healthy for your heart. You will also learn the benefits of consuming more natural nutrient-rich whole foods, and you will be introduced to healthy whole-food-based diets such as the raw food movement, juicing and blending, and much more.

Nutrition is an important part of a healthy lifestyle. Nowadays, we are more aware of the importance of proper daily nutrition, which has recently become a core component of modern medical practice. Until recently, medical schools taught very few courses in nutrition.

A vital component of a healthy heart and longevity is a well-balanced diet.

Considering my own experience, I can honestly say that medical students often graduate and become doctors with only a basic sense of how nutrition plays a role in maintaining good overall health. Without proper nutrition, one does not have enough energy to make it through the day and one's overall health declines, making one more susceptible to illness and disease.

In today's fast-paced world, so many things vie for our attention: jobs, school, kids, bills—and the list continues. Combine that with a lack of cooking skills and a habitual appetite for unhealthy fast foods, and we forget that we eat first and foremost for our nutritional health and to sustain our bodies, rather than as a matter of convenience.

We have replaced the value of fresh fruits and vegetables with the convenience of fast food. We eat at restaurants because it's easy to do so, never realizing that many of the foods served are not fresh but processed—frozen, freeze-dried, and dehydrated. Even at home, we sometimes feed ourselves and our families processed and pre-packaged foods. But at what cost?

Processed foods can affect almost every organ in the body and can prevent the body from being able to handle stress from illness, injury, surgery, childbirth, and many other activities of daily living. Much of the nutritional value of food is lost when it is processed and packaged. These processes significantly decrease the nutritional content of the foods.

Many doctors agree that processed foods are in large part responsible for type 2 diabetes, obesity, heart disease, high blood pressure, and even cancer and myriad additional health ailments. Currently, obesity in the United States and worldwide is reaching epidemic proportions, with more than one billion overweight or obese people and counting.

The statistics are even more staggering for our children. An estimated twenty-two million children under five are overweight worldwide.

According to the US Surgeon General, in the United States since 1980 the number of overweight children has doubled and the number of overweight adolescents has tripled.

What are the consequences?

The CDC estimates that one out of three children born in 2000 will develop type 2 diabetes in his or her lifetime, and that children born in 2000 may not outlive their parents. The incidences of type 2 diabetes have tripled in the last thirty years. Our children are at risk of developing more co-morbidities associated with obesity, such as high blood pressure, high cholesterol, diabetes, heart disease, strokes, certain cancers, sleep apnea, osteoarthritis, gallbladder disease, gastro-esophageal reflux disease, and gout, not to mention the psychological and emotional effects of obesity.

Research is also linking poor dietary habits to dramatic effects on the brain, including an increase in violent behavior. One out of every eight deaths in America is caused by an illness directly related to being overweight or obese. The cost of obesity and its related diseases to the healthcare industry is in the billions of dollars and is outstripping our health-care resources.

Being the mother of three school-aged children—thirteen-year-old Jonathan, ten-year-old Sarah, and nine-year-old Andrew at the time of this writing—I am particularly sensitive to this issue. Parental ignorance cannot be deemed an excuse for our negligent behaviors. As parents, we are in total control of our children's oral intake, at least during their early formative years.

Allowing our children to overindulge in junk food, sodas, and other foods totally devoid of any nutritional value while not

The CDC estimates that one out of three children born in 2000 will develop type 2 diabetes in his or her lifetime, and that children born in 2000 may not outlive their parents.

> Your body is a finely tuned machine, and it should be revered and maintained. The body's natural state is to be healthy, and it will move itself in that direction as long as we don't impede the process.

encouraging a healthy intake of fresh fruits and vegetables borders on child abuse or neglect when one considers the dire consequences of these actions. By ignoring the hazards of these poor food choices and allowing obesity, diabetes, and high cholesterol to set in early, we place our children in harm's way for the development of heart disease, cancer, arthritis, a poor quality of life, and a shorter lifespan.

As such, this is my challenge and my call to action—we need to take a closer look at ourselves and the way we live, and how we feed our families. Our children are depending on us to model healthy behaviors. With knowledge, education, and support, we can change the future of our lives and those of our children.

I developed my nonprofit organization, Revitalize Youth (www.revitalizeyouth.org), to address the issue of childhood obesity and to provide education on nutrition, exercise, and the importance of a healthy mind-body connection in our school districts. Some of the proceeds from this book will go directly to fund this project, which is a passion of mine. Additional proceeds will benefit the Alliance for a Healthier Generation, a nonprofit organization founded by the AHA and the Clinton Foundation.

The Alliance works to reduce the prevalence of childhood obesity and to empower kids to develop lifelong, healthy habits. The Alliance works with schools, companies, community organizations, health-care professionals, and families to transform the conditions and systems that lead to healthier children. To learn more and join the movement, visit www.HealthierGeneration.org.

Your body is a finely tuned machine, and it should be revered and maintained. The body's natural state is to be healthy, and it will move itself in that direction as long as we don't impede the process. Food is our fuel source. We eat for pleasure, but our bodies eat for nutrients. Nutrients sustain life and allow us to grow and stay healthy, beautiful, and strong.

You can save your body energy by eating more wholesome, natural foods. The less energy your body spends on digestion and breaking down unhealthy processed foods devoid of nutritional value, the more energy it will retain. Doctors and nutrition experts recommend that 70 percent of your diet should consist of fruits and vegetables. The remaining 30 percent should include healthy whole grains, animal or vegetarian proteins, and healthy fats. Choose a diet that will optimize your health.

WHOLE FOODS

Whole foods are foods that have not been refined or processed in any way. They are foods that can be consumed in their natural state, such as whole grains, fruits, vegetables, beans, nuts, seeds, wild-caught or sustainably farmed seafood, organically raised (hormone- and antibiotic-free) meat, organic unprocessed dairy products, and free-range eggs.

Whole foods mobilize and increase amino acids, the building blocks of protein. They also provide fuel for energy production, maintain resistance to stresses such as infections and disease, and promote happy personalities and emotional stability.

Whole foods do not contain preservatives. When food is processed or refined, many nutrients are often lost or purposely removed. In addition, food processing involves adding artificial ingredients, preservatives, chemicals, trans fats, salt, and sugar. These additives are bad for you; they interfere with your digestive system and prevent the arteries from producing nitric oxide. Nitric oxide helps to protect the arteries from a buildup of LDL cholesterol, which can cause blockages and ruptures that often result in heart attacks and strokes.

Processed foods are also very difficult for the body to digest, and they can contribute to weight gain, digestive problems, increased blood sugar levels, and high blood pressure. Therefore, experts suggest that for optimal heart health, minimally 70 to 80 percent and optimally 100 percent of our diet should be made up of whole foods.

THE RAW FOOD MOVEMENT

The raw food diet has become very popular with people around the world due to its many benefits for overall health. The diet is based on the idea that several foods lose a great deal of their nutritional value when they are exposed to heat. Raw food enthusiasts ensure that whole foods that have not been heated above 115 degrees Fahrenheit compose at least 75 percent of their daily diet.

A study at the German Institute of Human Nutrition revealed that people who included raw plant foods as 70 to 100 percent of their diet showed significant decreases in LDL cholesterol and triglyceride levels.

Raw foods aid in cleansing the bloodstream, which allows better blood flow to the heart. In addition, a raw food diet is good for you because it is very low in total fat, cholesterol, sugar, and salt, plus high in vitamins, minerals, and phytochemicals.

Such a diet has many benefits for the heart and overall well-being. It can lower cholesterol and blood sugar, promote weight loss, improve rheumatologic conditions, boost the immune system, and protect against cancer due to the high antioxidant content of the food. The only current concern is that it may be difficult to get a sufficient amount of protein, calcium, vitamin D, and vitamin B12 from a strictly raw food diet.

COOKING METHODS

While consuming foods in their raw, natural whole state is ideal for maximum nutrient value, many people are not able to tolerate this form of intake. If one needs to heat the food, then cooking time and temperature play a vital role in determining nutrient loss. The water-soluble vitamins B, C, and folate are most affected. As such, limiting the amount of water with which you cook your vegetables also plays a key factor in nutrient loss.

Steaming, quick stir-frying, and even microwave cooking—due to its short cooking time and use of minimal water—are effective ways to preserve nutrients. However, I am not a proponent of microwave cooking, as I question the effects that microwave emission heating can have on the stability of food molecules, which could in turn have questionable biological effects on our bodies.

Some preparation methods to consider are cooking vegetables al dente, covering the pot to retain steam and limit overall cooking time, using low heat, repurposing the leftover cooking water into soup or sauce, and using as little water as possible or investing in a waterless cooking system, such as Saladmaster.

Cookware that allows for cooking without oil is another great investment in your health. Whenever possible, use vegetable broth as a base for stir-frying your vegetables. By avoiding the consumption of animal protein, you will almost eliminate the need for oil.

However, if you do need to use oil, consider working with grapeseed oil for its high heat stability. All other liquid oils have a lower heating point and turn rancid, leading to oxidative stress in the body when they are heated and consumed. Coconut oil and palm oil, which also have high heat stability, are saturated fats and will raise cholesterol levels.

MEAT AND DAIRY PRODUCTS

The *Journal of Internal Medicine* recently published a report about the long-term effects of red meat consumption, and the results did not bode well for heart health.

In the study, scientists followed over 120,000 people for twenty-eight years, taking note of their diet and meat consumption. It was discovered that people who ate red meat on a regular basis had an 18 percent higher chance of dying of heart disease, and a 10 percent higher risk of developing cancer. Moreover, people who consumed large amounts of processed meats, such as sausages, bacon, and salami, increased their chances of dying from heart disease by 21 percent, and their risk of dying of cancer by 16 percent.

This study prompted the World Cancer Research Fund to issue a statement urging people to avoid processed meats and to limit their red meat intake to 500 grams a week.

Many of us have been raised to believe that milk and dairy products are good for our health, primarily as sources of protein and calcium. However, studies show that dairy products can contribute to cardiovascular problems as well as heartburn, stomach pains, diarrhea, and excess gas. Dairy products are often high in saturated fats and cholesterol, which wreak havoc on the cardiovascular system.

In addition, research shows that there is a correlation between milk consumption and type 1 diabetes. In 2001, the Finnish journal *Diabetologica* published a study that showed that infants with a genetic predisposition to diabetes increased their risk of developing the disease if they were fed cow's milk early in life.

Research also shows that, contrary to popular belief, milk does not make our bones stronger or stave off osteoporosis. Countries that have the highest consumption of dairy (United States, England, and Sweden) also have the highest incidence of osteoporosis, whereas countries such as China and Japan, where the consumption of animal protein and dairy is low, have a low incidence of osteoporosis. Instead of dairy, a healthy diet of whole grains, fruit, and vegetables and plenty of exercise are key to healthy bones and healthy hearts.

Although our bodies are designed to consume and digest meat and dairy products, animal proteins are not necessary for a healthy diet. Some people find that by simply eliminating meat and dairy from their diet, they feel healthier and more energetic, and they exhibit fewer signs of illness. A vegetarian or vegan diet can be extremely beneficial to your health.

However, some people find that they still crave steak, chicken, fish, milk, and cheeses. Experts believe that these cravings stem from a lack of vitamins and proteins in the body. For example, if you are craving meat, you may have low protein levels. Likewise, if you crave dairy products, you may be suffering from a lack of calcium, vitamin A, or vitamin D in your body. If you want to eat healthier, try replacing meat and dairy products with high-protein foods like quinoa, avocados, peanut butter, chickpeas, or oats.

If you absolutely cannot go without meat or dairy, look for natural grain-fed animal products that have not been injected with hormones, lean meats such as poultry and fish, and low-fat or nonfat dairy products.

A DRASTIC IMPROVEMENT

I had a patient, Tony, who like many people paid little attention to his diet. He simply ate what he liked, whenever he felt like it. Although he would occasionally eat fruits and vegetables, a large part of his diet was made up of red meat, pasta, cheeses, and processed foods. In addition, his fast-paced and stressful career left him with little time to exercise or relax.

On a rare day off in 2008, Tony was walking his dog when he began to have intense chest pains. He was diagnosed with angina as a result of atherosclerosis. He underwent an angioplasty, where a balloon catheter was inserted into his blocked artery to inflate the artery and allow for more blood flow to his heart. He was also prescribed a number of medications including beta-blockers and vitamins.

This was a real wake-up call for Tony. Although he was only fifty-one years old, his unhealthy diet, lack of exercise, and stressful lifestyle had contributed to high cholesterol and high blood pressure. His lifestyle had led to blocked arteries, a condition that could have resulted in a heart attack or stroke.

Because of this frightening event, Tony made the decision to start eating better and began to incorporate healthy whole foods into his daily diet. He started eating more fresh vegetables and fruits, whole grains, and lean meats. He cut out as many unhealthy processed foods from his diet as he could and avoided red meat and dairy products. Tony also began to exercise on a daily basis and made a concerted effort to take more time off work and relax.

Today, Tony is thirty-five pounds lighter, and he says he feels healthier and more energetic than when he was in his thirties. To date, he has not suffered another cardiac episode.

His story is just one of many where patients see drastic improvements in their health after switching to a healthier eating plan, exercising regularly, and cutting down on stress.

JUICING

One quick and easy way to meet the nutrient requirement is by juicing fresh vegetables and fruits. Juicing removes the fibers and solid materials in foods so that you are left with pure, nutritious juice in its natural state.

The vitamins and minerals in juices are easily absorbed by your body, as you do not need to use valuable energy digesting the fiber in the skin or flesh of the plants. This aids in cell growth and rejuvenates your organs, such as your heart, lungs, and kidneys. Moreover, the nutrients in juices help your body to heal itself, which makes juicing ideal for people who are recovering from illnesses or surgery.

Drinking pure juices flushes your digestive tract, which can strengthen your internal organs and help you lose weight. Obesity and excessive weight are major contributors to cardiovascular disease and diabetes.

Weight gain results from a poor diet that relies largely on high-caloric processed foods. It is very difficult for your body to digest processed foods, so residue from these foods often gets stuck in your digestive tract. This buildup of residue can cause you to crave more unhealthy foods and feel sluggish and unhealthy. Fresh, nutritious juice contains live plant enzymes that help cleanse your body by flushing out indigestible food residue, and thereby increasing your energy levels and giving you a greater sense of wellness.

Another healthy advantage of juicing is that it can clear your blood of free radicals. These are the dead cells in your bloodstream that have no electrical charge. They often attach themselves to the healthy, living cells in your body, which may cause cancerous growths, poorly functioning organs, and premature aging.

The healthy compounds in juices called antioxidants can help to eliminate free radicals from your bloodstream so that your body operates at

To get the maximum amount of vitamins and minerals, focus on taking in a rainbow spectrum of different colors of fruits and vegetables, paying particular attention to dense, dark colors.

optimal health. People who drink fresh fruit and vegetable juices on a regular basis often have increased metabolism and get sick less often than people who do not include healthy juices in their diet.

It should be noted that even if you drink a significant amount of juice, you should still include whole fruits and vegetables in your diet for the fiber that they offer. Fruits and some vegetables are very high in natural sugars. The natural fiber within fruits and vegetables keeps their caloric density low and helps with satiety, thereby preventing the overconsumption of calories.

People with diabetes and those struggling with their weight should be careful about the types and amount of juice they consume. In particular, carrot juice and beetroot juice contain high levels of sugar.

BLENDING

Blending is another way to introduce more fruits and vegetables in your diet. When you blend foods, you break down the food so that the water and enzymes are released and you are left with the vitamins, minerals, and healthy compounds in the pulp and flesh of the plant materials. Unlike a juicer, a blender does not remove the skin and flesh of the fruits and vegetables, thereby providing fiber.

Although your body does need to use energy to break down the fibers in the blended foods, the blender does most of the difficult work, making it easier to digest the foods. This is ideal for people who are healing from an illness or injury. In addition, your body needs a certain amount of fiber to function properly and ward off disease. Fiber acts like a broom in your digestive system, cleansing your internal system and helping to regulate digestion. Not only that, but fiber helps to keep you full for a longer period of time.

Therefore, blending fruits and vegetables would be ideal for meal replacements, keeping you satisfied for up to two to four hours after having a healthy blended smoothie. According to the Mayo Clinic, eating a diet high in fiber can reduce your risk of heart disease, stroke, and diabetes.

Blending is an excellent way to boost your immune system and introduce more healthy plant material into your diet. When you eat blended foods, it is very easy for your body to absorb the vitamins, minerals, and phytochemicals that are in the fruits and vegetables, as much of the cell wall has been broken. These nutrients can lower your blood pressure and LDL (the bad type of cholesterol), while increasing your levels of HDL (the good type of cholesterol). Moreover, the nutrients and phytochemicals in fresh, blended fruits and vegetables can regulate your blood sugars. This reduces your risk of developing diabetes, hypertension, and cardiovascular disease.

THE RAINBOW SPECTRUM

More important than the method of preparation of the fruits and vegetables is the quantity and quality of the produce. To get the maximum amount of vitamins and minerals, focus on taking in a rainbow spectrum of different colors of fruits and vegetables, paying particular attention to dense, dark colors:

- Red produce provides vitamin A (beta carotene), vitamin C, manganese, fiber, and lycopene, which has cancer-fighting properties.

- Orange produce provides vitamins A, C, and B6, as well as potassium and fiber.

- Yellow produce, such as bananas, provides potassium, fiber, manganese, vitamin A, and magnesium.

- Green produce provides a host of vitamins and minerals, including lutein, which aids eyesight, and folate, which promotes cellular reproduction.

- Blue produce, such as blueberries, is loaded with antioxidants and fiber.

- Purple produce provides anthocyanin, a powerful antioxidant for the blood vessels and skin, as well as vitamin A and flavonoids.

- White produce, such as cauliflower, rutabagas, and parsnips, provides vitamins C, K, and folate, whereas onion and garlic provide allicin for heart and blood-vessel protection.

ORGANIC VERSUS CONVENTIONAL

It is commonly believed that organic foods provide a higher nutrient content and therefore are healthier than their conventional counterparts.

However, a systematic review published in the September 2009 issue of the *American Journal of Clinical Nutrition* and a more recent Stanford study do not support this commonly held belief. There was a lower nitrogen and higher phosphorous content in organic produce, but contents of vitamin C, calcium, potassium, soluble solids, copper, iron, nitrates, manganese, ash, specific proteins, sodium, carbohydrates, β-carotene, and sulfur did not differ. Organic produce had a 30 percent lower risk of having pesticide contamination, which is significant considering the neurogenic and estrogenic effects of pesticides.

The results of the Stanford study have met with great controversy, as they contradict conventional wisdom. Kirsten Brandt of Newcastle University, who conducted a similar review of the relevant studies in 2011, reported the opposite conclusion: that organics carried far more of the heart-healthy nutrients and flavanols than conventional foods.

The United States Environmental Protection Agency (EPA) notes that laboratory studies show that pesticides can cause health problems, such as birth defects, nerve damage, cancer, and other effects that might occur over a long period of time, depending on the toxicity of the pesticide and the quantity consumed. Pesticides pose a unique health risk to children due to children's developing nature, higher consumption of food relative to their body weight, and certain behaviors that increase their risk of pesticide exposure.

The serious pesticide risk is the neurogenical and estrogenic properties of the pesticides, which can lead to increased cancer risk and degenerative neurological conditions. In addition, the benefit of consuming

DIRTY DOZEN AND THE CLEAN 15 LIST

Despite the recent Stanford study, I believe it is still prudent to make individualized decisions when it comes to your family's food source. Given the increased expense and limited availability of buying organic, it might be worthwhile to consider the Dirty Dozen and Clean 15 List published by the Environmental Working Group each year. A recent Dirty Dozen list of produce includes apples, celery, sweet bell peppers, peaches, strawberries, nectarines (imported), grapes, spinach, lettuce, cucumbers, blueberries (domestic), and potatoes. An updated Clean 15 list of produce that can be purchased conventionally includes onions, sweet corn, pineapples, avocados, cabbage, sweet peas, asparagus, mangoes, eggplants, kiwis, cantaloupes (domestic), sweet potatoes, grapefruits, watermelons, and mushrooms.

organic products is to ensure against genetically modified products and the deleterious health effects discussed below.

GENETICALLY MODIFIED ORGANISMS (GMOS)

Even though genetically modified products have been on the market for only twenty years, it is estimated that over 70 percent of all items in American food stores contain genetically modified organisms (GMOs). Genetically engineered plants and animals are created by taking the genetic material of one organism and inserting it permanently into the genetic code of another organism. Currently, between 80 and 90 percent of all US corn, soybeans, canola, and cotton are genetically produced.

Much of this industry is unregulated, and there have been many claims that the political and financial structure has led unsuspecting consumers to purchase unlabeled GMO products despite findings that such foods may pose serious health risks. Potential hazards include toxicity, infertility, genetic birth defects, infant mortality, autism, allergenicity, asthma, antibiotic resistance, immune suppression, autoimmune diseases, diabetes, and cancer.

Many nations require the labeling of GMO products, led by Europe in 1998 and followed by Japan, Australia, and New Zealand in 2001; China, Saudi Arabia, and South Korea in 2002; Thailand and Indonesia in 2003; Brazil and Venezuela in 2004; Taiwan in 2005; Russia, India, and Chile in 2006; and finally South Africa in 2011. However, regulators in the United States and Canada still keep their consumers ignorant about their food supply.

The nonprofit Institute of Responsible Technology provides a free iPhone app, ShopNoGMO, which gives consumers a handy resource to identify non-GMO-brand choices. One can also look for specific labeling identifying non-GMO products. For produce, look at the four- or five-digit number on the label: a four-digit number indicates conventionally grown produce which may or may not be genetically modified. A five-digit label beginning with a numeral 8 signifies a GMO product. However, not all GMOs are identified as such, because this labeling method is optional. A five-digit number beginning with a numeral 9 indicates that the food is organically grown and therefore not a GMO.

Jeffrey Smith's 2003 *Seeds of Deception* and Bill Engdahl's 2007 *Seeds of Destruction: The Hidden Agenda of Genetic Manipulation* are two interesting reads on the subject. *Genetic Roulette*, a well-produced documentary on this topic, is another good resource if you're interested in learning more.

PHYTOCHEMICALS

Phytochemicals are natural compounds found in plants such as fruits and vegetables. They protect the plants from bacteria, fungi, viruses, and pests. These natural chemicals also give plants their bright colors, flavors, and odors. The more colorful, flavorful, or strongly scented a plant is, the higher the concentration of phytochemicals.

These chemicals are very beneficial for humans because they act as antioxidants, antibacterials, antivirals, and anti-inflammatories in the body. They boost our immune systems, regulate hormones and sugar levels, lower cholesterol, slow the aging process, and protect against heart disease, stroke, diabetes, cancer, and osteoporosis. Thousands of phyto-chemicals are found in the foods we eat, and these compounds assist in keeping us healthy and warding off disease.

CAROTENOIDS

Carotenoids are phytochemicals that act as antioxidants in the body, elimi-nating free radicals and promoting optimal health. They can be found in bright yellow, orange, and red foods, as well as leafy green vegetables. Foods that contain carotenoids can lower your risk of heart disease, high blood pressure, and certain types of cancer. Some of the more common types of carotenoids include beta-carotene, lycopene, and xanthophylls.

Beta-Carotene

Beta-carotene can be found in red and orange foods such as carrots, red bell peppers, oranges, and grapefruit, as well as in spinach and kale. This powerful phytochemical lowers bad LDL cholesterol, which in turn reduces the likelihood of plaque building up on the artery walls. This improves blood flow and lowers the risk of a heart attack. Studies show that beta-carotene may also lower your risk of developing lung cancer.

Lycopene

Lycopene is a powerful antioxidant that can be found in red foods such as tomatoes, watermelons, and red bell peppers. This carotenoid can protect the arteries from damage, reduce inflammation, and prevent LDL cholesterol from oxidizing. This helps to protect you against coronary heart disease and stroke. In a study by the Harvard School of Medicine, women who consumed lycopene on a regular basis had 50 percent less chance of developing heart disease over a five-year period.

Xanthophylls

Xanthophylls are a form of carotenoids that include lutein, cryptozanthin, and zeaxanthin. They can be found in yellow and orange foods such as corn, squash, egg yolks, and carrots, as well as in broccoli, spinach, kale, avocados, and green peas. They are anti-inflammatory and anti-aging, and they protect the body against free radicals and atherosclerosis.

Xanthophylls also help your body to convert vitamin A to retinol, which helps protect the eyes from harmful UV rays.

POLYPHENOLS

Polyphenols act as antioxidants to protect your body from free-radical activity and prevent inflammation that can aggravate coronary heart disease. These phytochemicals ward off cardiovascular disease and cancer, and they encourage healthy gastrointestinal and urinary tract function. They can be found in many different foods including honey, green tea, red wine, strawberries, plums, and olive oil.

ANTHOCYANINS AND FLAVONOLS

These phytochemicals are powerful antioxidants found in a wide variety of fruits and vegetables including berries, apples, jalapeño peppers, eggplants, cherries, and grape seeds. Research shows that anthocyanins and flavonols are effective in protecting against heart disease, diabetes, and certain types of cancer. They also have an anti-inflammatory effect and can slow the aging process.

HEART-HEALTHY SUPERFOODS

The ideal diet for a healthy heart should include a wide range of foods such as whole grains, legumes, vegetables, fruits, and healthy proteins. While most fresh, whole foods have a very positive effect on your health, vitality, and well-being, research shows that certain foods are better for your cardiovascular system than others. The following list includes foods known to positively affect heart health.

GREENS

Raw green leafy vegetables are the most nutrient-packed, calorie-poor foods available. Greens are rich in folate, a B complex essential for cellular growth and reproduction. They provide valuable vitamins (K, C, E, B) and minerals (iron, calcium, potassium, magnesium). Greens are rich in phytonutrients, including beta carotene, lutein, and zeaxanthin. Greens even contain a small amount of omega-3 fatty acids. Eating great quantities of green leafy vegetables is a great way to lose weight, as they have very few carbohydrates, and the carbs are fiber dense, limiting the impact on blood sugar.

CRUCIFEROUS VEGETABLES

Cruciferous vegetables flower in the shape of a cross, hence their name. This group of vegetables has been studied extensively for its life-giving properties, including the prevention of cancer, cardiovascular disease, and diabetes.

Cruciferous vegetables contain glucosinolates, which convert to isothiocyanates when their cell walls are broken down by chopping, blending, or chewing. These isothiocyanates have potent anti-cancer effects, reduce inflammation, and diminish oxidative stress. In addition, these vegetables supply the body with essential nutrients, including vitamins, soluble fiber, minerals, essential fats, carbohydrates, and protein. Cruciferous vegetables lose a great deal of nutrients when they are exposed to high heat, so it is best to lightly steam or sauté these vegetables to preserve their healthy value.

BERRIES

Berries are truly superfoods: they have amazing taste and brilliant colors, and they are packed full of flavonoids, including anthocyanins. Numerous researchers have shown the cardioprotective effects of berries through the lowering of blood pressure, the reduction in oxidative stress, the reduction in inflammation, and the beneficial effects on cholesterol. This translates into a greater than 30 percent decrease in the risk of heart attacks with just three servings of berries a week.

WHOLE GRAINS

According to the AHA, adults should eat between six and eight servings of grains a day. Ideally they should all be whole grains. Grains supply your body with vital dietary fiber and can lower your cholesterol.

A Nurses' Health Study at Harvard showed that women who managed to incorporate two to three servings of whole grains into their diets lowered their risk of heart attacks, type 2 diabetes, and heart disease by 30 percent when compared to women who only ate one serving of whole grains a day. You can get whole grains from cereals, breads, and rice.

LEGUMES, SEEDS, AND NUTS

Seeds, nuts, and legumes are great options for getting a decent amount of protein without consuming animal products. These healthy whole foods are rich in protein, fiber, and essential amino acids and monounsaturated fats. A study by the University of Minnesota analyzed the eating habits of more than twelve thousand middle-aged men in sixteen countries. It showed that the people who included a generous amount of legumes (at least one cup daily) in their diets had a jaw-dropping 82 percent lower risk of developing coronary heart disease.

A more recent study published in the *Journal of Internal Medicine* showed that legumes improved type 2 diabetic patients' glycemic control (level of blood sugar), improved blood pressure, and lowered heart-disease risk. The effects of nuts and seeds on diet has also been studied extensively, and the experts say that adding these foods to your diet can also lower your risk for heart disease. In addition, nuts, seeds, and legumes can be eaten on their own as a tasty snack, or mixed into salads, stir-fries, soups, and sauces for a wholesome and healthy meal.

HEART-HEALTHY FISH

Fish is an excellent source of protein that is light, tasty, and good for the heart. Many of my patients want to eat healthier, but they are not ready to commit to a vegetarian or vegan diet. To these patients, I suggest replacing red meat and poultry with healthy whole fish and seafood.

However, not all types of fish and seafood are good for the body. The AHA suggests eating two to three servings a week of fish that are high in omega-3 fatty acids, such as salmon, halibut, and trout. In addition, the healthiest way to prepare fish is by baking, steaming, or grilling the fish rather than frying it in oil. You can add a squeeze of lemon or healthy herbs to season.

I will provide a word of caution, however, regarding the source of your fish. It is often the case that, when demand is increased, unethical and unscrupulous practices come into play and taint the source of the supply of the food in question.

Fish farming is common practice, and now most of the salmon consumed and sold in grocery stores and at restaurants is farm raised. High-density overcrowding, unsanitary and inhumane conditions, contaminated fish feeds, overuse of antibiotics and steroids, and bacterial, parasitic, and lice infections produce highly stressed and unhealthy, possibly diseased fish, which are then dyed with food coloring to improve their appearance.

A comprehensive study of farmed versus wild salmon, published in the January 2004 issue of Science, found a significantly higher level of cancer-causing and other health-related contaminants in farm-raised salmon as compared to wild-caught salmon. Another study commissioned by the Environmental Working Group (EWG) found contamination of polychlorinated biphenyl (PCB) fourteen times greater in farm-raised versus wild salmon.

PCB is a persistent, cancer-causing chemical that was banned in the United States in 1976, but it continues to contaminate the environment and our food supply. If the level of PCB discovered in this study of farmed salmon was found in the wild, the EPA fish advisory would recommend the consumption of no more than one salmon meal a month. The EPA standards for PCB levels are five hundred times more protective than the PCB limits applied by the FDA to commercially sold fish, according to the EWG.

Thus it is advisable to consult guides such as the Monterey Bay Aquarium Seafood Watch when buying salmon. These guides provide the latest information on the sustainable seafood choices that are available in different regions of the United States.

For those wishing to avoid fish altogether, excellent non-animal sources of omega-3 include ground flaxseeds and hemp seeds, along with grapeseed oil, olive oil, tofu, walnuts, and to a lesser degree, dark leafy greens.

OTHER HEART-HEALTHY FOODS

DARK CHOCOLATE

Chocolate is one sweet that not only tastes good, but is also good for your heart. Research shows that chocolate containing 70 percent cacao or more can regulate your blood pressure and hormones, thin the blood so you are at lower risk of blood clots that can cause heart attacks, and battle inflammation. Furthermore, antioxidants in dark chocolate can fight harmful free radicals in the body. For the maximum health benefit, raw cacao (more on this later) should be consumed rather than the chocolate processed with sugar and dairy.

HONEY

This rich, amber-colored natural sweetener not only tastes good, but it is also great for your cardiovascular system. Honey is antibacterial and antifungal, meaning it fights off harmful elements in the body that can cause illness. Studies show that honey can also lower bad LDL cholesterol and C-reactive protein levels, both of which are precursors to coronary heart disease.

Moreover, honey is highly effective in controlling blood sugar levels and aiding the body's resistance to insulin. People with diabetes seem to be able to tolerate honey much better than refined sugars, making honey a healthy alternative to sucrose. Honey contains flavonoids, antioxidants that ward off certain cancers and heart disease. Honey in combination with cinnamon consumed daily reduces cholesterol, strengthens the blood vessels and the heartbeat, and lowers the risk of heart attacks.

OLIVE OIL

Olive oil is a huge component of the Mediterranean diet, which is known to have cardiovascular benefits. Studies show that extra-virgin olive oil can significantly lower your risk for cardiovascular disease. In addition, this tasty and light oil is high in monounsaturated fats, which can lower dangerous levels of cholesterol in the body.

Moreover, olive oil—despite its high calorie content—can regulate insulin and blood sugar levels, prevent blood clotting, lower blood pressure, and reduce obesity. It strengthens the immune system and has anti-inflammatory and anti-cancer properties due to its high level of antioxidants, in the form of polyphenols. If you want to boost your cardiovascular system and improve your overall health, incorporate olive oil into your diet.

Note, however, that olive oil is meant to be consumed cold-pressed and should not be heated. While it is clearly a preferred source of healthy fat compared to meat consumption, supporters of whole foods will argue for the consumption of olives, although olives are too bitter to be eaten raw and need to undergo a curing process, which depletes them of some of their polyphenols.

WHEATGRASS

Wheatgrass is typically squeezed for its juice, which is rich in nutrients and heart-healthy compounds. Researchers believe that the high levels of chlorophyll in wheatgrass enable oxygen to flow to the heart more easily through the bloodstream. In addition, vitamins and minerals such as vitamin A, vitamin C, vitamin E, magnesium, calcium, and iron help to ease pressure on the blood vessels and prevent plaque buildup in the arteries, which reduces the risk of heart disease and stroke.

HERBS FOR HEART HEALTH

Certain herbs have a very powerful effect on the body's immune system and can help to ward off disease, revitalize the cells, and promote efficient organ function. Both Eastern and Western medical traditions have relied on herbs for centuries to cure illnesses and strengthen the body's defenses against disease.

Although modern Western medical practice does not typically prescribe herbs as a form of treatment against disease, many doctors and nutritionists now see the value in specific plants and spices for medicinal treatments. Herbs have the benefit of being completely natural, and unlike biomedicine, many herbs produce little to no side effects. Moreover, herbs can be added to food to enhance the flavor of dishes and promote heart health. However, as with any medicine, it is important to discuss your particular medical condition with a doctor before incorporating herbs and spices into your diet.

EASTERN HERBS

Eastern medical practitioners have used herbs for centuries to treat cardio-vascular problems and encourage healthy heart function. Both Traditional Chinese Medicine (TCM) and Ayurvedic medicine rely on a number of herbal remedies to treat heart palpitations, poor circulation, chest pains, irregular heart rates, blocked arteries, high cholesterol and blood pressure, heart attacks, and strokes.

In TCM, it is believed that heart problems result when the meridians in the body are blocked so that qi, or life energy, cannot flow properly. TCM practitioners believe that certain herbs can be used to remove blockages and encourage efficient circulation.

Ayurvedic medicine also focuses on the flow of energy through merid-ians, as well as the powerful connection between the mind and body. For centuries, Ayurvedic doctors have been aware of the positive effects that some plants have on energy levels, circulation, emotional health, and vital organ function. Eastern herbs are typically prescribed in their natural state either in tea or capsule form.

While you may be able to find Asian herbs such as garlic and ginger in your local supermarket, others may be a bit more elusive. A TCM practitioner or an Ayurvedic doctor will likely have access to many different beneficial herbs, and he or she can prescribe safe dosages for your particular health condition. You can also find many herbal remedies online, although I strongly advise against self-medicating.

If you buy herbs online, you need to be very careful about seeking out reputable sources. The Internet is rife with people trying to make quick money by selling counterfeit medicines that could cause serious health problems. I advise you to do your own research on this topic, as adequately covering it is beyond the scope of this book. While there are many authorities on the subject, one resource that I often turn to is George Mateljan's The World's Healthiest Foods (www.whfoods.org).

I will highlight one herb, turmeric, which my family regularly uses in cooking, for its cardiovascular benefits. A study published in the *American Journal of Cardiology* in 2011 found the administration of curcuminoids, the natural phenols found in turmeric, resulted in a 56 percent relative reduction of myocardial infarction (heart attack) after coronary artery bypass.

Another study published in *Nutrition Research* in 2012 found that curcumin, the primary polyphenol in turmeric, was just as effective in improving endothelial or vascular function as moderate aerobic exercise in post-menopausal women. The same research group in Japan published in the *American Journal of Hypertension* that combining daily curcumin with regular endurance exercise may reduce the stress on the heart (left ventricular afterload reduction).

The antioxidant and anti-inflammatory properties of curcumin are postulated to be the mechanisms behind the cardiovascular protection. In addition, curcumin has insulin-sensitizing effects, which can result in the dramatic lowering of triglyceride levels.

My recommendation is to take turmeric supplements over isolated curcumin for its more effective anti-inflammatory properties. The supplements should be standardized for 95 percent curcuminoids and should contain black pepper or piperine to help with absorption. As with all supplements, please consult your physician, especially if you are on prescription medication. If you cook with turmeric, add some black pepper to the food as well for better absorption.

WESTERN HERBS

Although modern Western medicine focuses on using pharmaceuticals to treat the symptoms of illness, herbal medicine has a long history in Western medical practice. The ancient Romans, Greeks, and Egyptians used herbs to prevent and treat disease, and today many Western herbalists also draw on this knowledge, as well as on TCM, Ayurvedic medicine, and Native American lore and plant remedies, to heal the body and protect against cardiovascular disease.

Many of the plants and herbs used in Western herbal remedies, such as garlic, ginger, and peppermint, can be found in your garden or at the supermarket.

LITTLE-KNOWN SUPERFOODS

It seems like every other day a story breaks about a new superfood on the market that can miraculously help you shed pounds, look younger, and feel fitter. While some of these miracle foods are undoubtedly nothing more than exotic fruits or seeds, a few have been scientifically proven to have major health benefits. The following are some little-known superfoods that can boost your immune system, strengthen the heart, and protect against cardiovascular disease.

CAMU CAMU

Camu camu is a tree fruit that grows in the Amazon region of South America. It looks similar to cherries and has a very sour taste. Despite its tart flavor, studies at the Instituto de Biotecnologia in Lima, Peru, revealed that the camu camu fruit is very high in vitamin C and antioxidants that can boost the immune system and protect against heart disease. Researchers also believe that consumption of this fruit may be effective in preventing certain types of cancer.

CHILEAN MAQUI BERRY

The native Mapuche people in Chile have been eating the maqui berry for centuries for its health-boosting properties. Studies show that these small berries contain very high levels of anthocyanins, which help to reduce inflammation and prevent cholesterol from oxidizing in the blood vessels. This reduces the risk of heart attacks and strokes. In addition, Chilean maqui berries can regulate blood glucose levels, which is good for preventing and treating diabetes.

ACAI BERRY

The small purple berries of the acai palm tree were once only consumed by tribes in the Amazon, but today they are sought out around the globe for their high levels of nutrients and antioxidants. Acai berries contain plenty of fiber, essential fatty acids, calcium, and phytochemicals such as anthocyanins and flavonoids. These phytochemicals aid in strengthening the heart by improving blood circulation, reducing tension on the blood vessels, and preventing atherosclerosis.

GOJI BERRIES

Goji berries are vibrant reddish-orange berries that grow in Asia and parts of southeastern Europe. Studies show that the berries contain very high levels of vitamins, minerals, essential fatty acids, and carotenoids. The antioxidant and anti-inflammatory properties of these nutrients work together to fight off diseases such as cancer, heart disease, hypertension, and diabetes. The berries can be consumed fresh and dried, and in soups, tea, or even wine.

SPIRULINA

This blue-green algae is a true superfood, as it contains myriad nutrients that are essential for optimal health. Spirulina is high in vitamins B12, C, D, A, and E, as well as protein, potassium, iron, zinc, and calcium. This potent combination of nutrients can lower blood pressure and bad LDL cholesterol, promote good circulation, strengthen the walls of the blood vessels, and prevent plaque buildup in the arteries. This helps to fight heart disease and improves cardiovascular function.

PURE CACAO POWDER

Sure, chocolate may be delicious and can even provide cardiovascular benefits, but a dark chocolate bar has nothing on pure cacao powder. When consumed in its pure, natural state, cacao powder can protect you from heart disease, diabetes, and stroke.

Pure cacao powder contains magnesium, which helps to regulate the levels of insulin in the bloodstream. In addition, this tasty powder is full of flavonoids that encourage the body to produce nitric oxide. This improves the elasticity of the blood vessels, allowing oxygen and blood to flow freely to the heart. Cacao contains a large concentration of antioxidants. It has theobromine, which acts as a mild stimulant and a diuretic, and phenyl-ethylamine, which is a mood enhancer. Raw cacao is loaded with essential vitamins (A, B1, B2, B3, C, E, and pantothenic acid) and essential minerals (magnesium, calcium, iron, zinc, copper, potassium, and manganese).

The next time you want a hot drink on a cold day, consider drinking cocoa made from pure cacao powder to protect your heart.

Many foods, herbs, and spices can help you to develop and maintain a healthy cardiovascular system. Whether you take up juicing, eat more whole foods in their natural states, or sprinkle your meals with heart-healthy herbs and spices, you will contribute to cleaner blood and arteries, better circulation, and improved heart function. This reduces your risk of heart attack, stroke, and diabetes.

The best part is that you do not have to drastically alter your diet to improve the condition of your heart and feel healthier, happier, and more energetic. Simply try adding a few of these superfoods into your meals, and you will do your heart a huge favor.

VITAMINS AND MINERALS FOR THE HEART

To prevent impurities from entering the body, it is important to eat a balanced diet of wholesome foods. Life in the twenty-first century is radically different from life even a hundred years ago. Many of the improvements have been for the betterment of society. However, one can argue that the removal of the simplicities of life has not necessarily benefited our bodies.

For example, our soil and the abundance of nutrients and minerals present in our natural food sources pales in comparison to what it was a

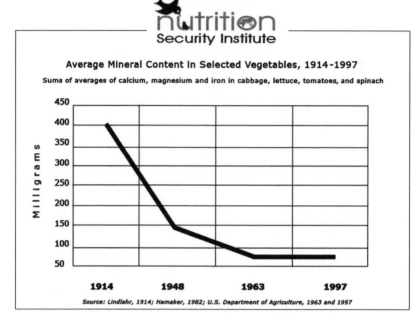

Fig. 3-1   Mineral Content of Vegetables

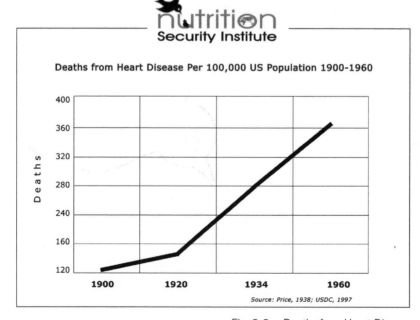

Fig. 3-2   Deaths from Heart Disease

hundred years ago. Our soil is the largest living component of our planet's biosphere, and the microbial life within our topsoil is the basis for the nutritional supply for all living organisms on the Earth. Yet the last five decades have witnessed significant destruction of this microbial ecosystem that exists within the topsoil, thanks to the arrival of inorganic fertilizers and the aggressive farming practices that have eroded our planet.

Figures 3-1 and 3-2 depict the tremendous rise in deaths from heart disease from 1900 to 1960 and the sharp decline in the mineral content of vegetables during a similar time period. While many factors contribute to the sharp rise in death from heart disease, certainly the increased consumption of processed foods and the general decline in both the intake of whole foods and the diminished nutritional and mineral contents of our food supply play a major role.

Numerous nutritional studies have linked many prevalent diseases to nutritional deficiencies. According to the United States Department of Agriculture (USDA), Americans as a whole lack the minerals calcium, magnesium, and potassium, as well as in the vitamins A, C, D, and E.

VITAMINS

Vitamins are essential organic compounds needed in the diet in small amounts to promote and regulate body functions and maintain good health. When vitamins are lacking in the diet, deficiency symptoms occur. Almost all foods contain certain vitamins; therefore it is important to eat a healthy, well-balanced diet daily.

B Vitamins

B vitamins are needed for internal energy production. Vitamins B12, B6, and B9 (folate) are known for their ability to

Numerous nutritional studies have linked many prevalent diseases to nutritional deficiencies.

combat cardiovascular disease. These vitamins help the body to convert homocysteine into methionine so that new proteins can be produced. Without the essential B vitamins, this reaction slows down and homocysteine levels in the body rise.

Scientists have discovered that homocysteine is directly linked to clogged arteries, or atherosclerosis. Some good sources of B vitamins include whole grains, leafy green vegetables, legumes, and seeds. Studies by the Harvard School of Public Health reveal that a diet rich in B vitamins can reduce the risk of heart disease, hypertension, and stroke. However, the benefits are not as high for people who have already suffered strokes and heart attacks.

Vitamin C

Most people only think of vitamin C (ascorbic acid) when they start noticing symptoms of a cold. Vitamin C functions as an antioxidant to protect against reactive oxygen molecules, and it not only boosts the immune system, but can also help lower the risk of heart disease, diabetes, hypertension, and blood clots.

Ascorbic acid reverses oxidation of cholesterol, which means you have less chance of developing atherosclerosis. In addition, it can lower high blood pressure, which protects the arteries from tension and stress. Moreover, vitamin C detoxifies histamine in the body, making it a natural antihistamine for those who have allergies.

The recommended dietary allowance (RDA) of vitamin C is 90 milligrams a day for men and 75 milligrams for women. This amount can easily be obtained by drinking an eight-ounce glass of orange juice daily. Cigarette smoking increases the recommended dietary intake of vitamin C because vitamin C is used to break down compounds taken into the body by cigarette smoke.

Citrus fruits such as oranges, lemons, and limes are an excellent source of vitamin C, as are strawberries, cantaloupes, and leafy greens and vegetables in the cabbage family.

Vitamin A

Vitamin A is important for vision. Are carrots really good for your eyes? The answer is yes, because carrots are high in vitamin A. Vitamin A deficiency is not common in developed countries; however, dietary intake surveys in the United States indicate that many Americans do not meet the daily recommendations. Dietary intakes below any RDA can be caused by poor food choices.

Vitamin D

Vitamin D is known as the sunshine vitamin. Enjoying the great outdoors is a great way to get some exercise and take in some vitamin D. This cardio-protective vitamin can be absorbed by the body from direct sun exposure.

Once vitamin D has been absorbed, it works to decrease levels of C-reactive protein, which is a risk factor for heart attacks. The vitamin also fights inflammation and insulin resistance, lowers high blood pressure, and strengthens the blood vessels and the heart. Scientists at Harvard discovered that men who took 600 IU (international units) of vitamin D a day reduced their risk of heart disease by 16 percent when compared to those who took 100 IU or less.

Vitamin D is important for heart health, but ingesting too much can have a negative effect. The maximum amount of vitamin D you should take in a day is 4,000 IU. A good ten minutes in the sun should do the trick. However, if you live in a climate with little sun, are above seventy years old, or have dark pigmentation, you may want to increase your intake of fatty fish, such as mackerel, salmon, tuna, or sardines. In addition, cod liver oil and some cereals contain high levels of vitamin D.

Vitamin E

Vitamin E is a powerful antioxidant that is found in nuts, seeds, oils, and leafy green vegetables. Antioxidants protect the body against free-radical damage, which is a major cause of cancer, atherosclerosis, and heart attacks. Studies show that vitamin E prevents LDL cholesterol from oxidizing. When LDL cholesterol oxidizes, it forms plaque on the lining of the arteries. This can cause blockages that prevent blood from flowing freely to the heart. Over time, a buildup of plaque can result in heart attacks and strokes.

The Cambridge Heart Antioxidant Study revealed that people who took vitamin E on a daily basis had 50 percent less chance of having a heart attack than people who did not take vitamin E. Some foods that are high in vitamin E include sunflower seeds and oil, avocados, spinach, broccoli, almonds, hazelnuts, and sweet potatoes.

Vitamin K2

Vitamin K2 is a fat-soluble vitamin that helps to regulate calcium levels in the body. This prevents against bone loss and the buildup of calcium in the arteries. In this way, vitamin K2 reduces your risk of atherosclerosis and coronary heart disease. In addition, it contributes to healthy bone growth.

Studies show people who have low levels of K2 have a much higher risk of developing cardiovascular disease. You can ensure that you are getting enough vitamin K2 by eating leafy green vegetables such as spinach, broccoli, cabbage, kale, and dandelion leaves.

Juice Plus+®

While getting an adequate amount of vitamins and nutrients is important, I am not a big proponent of synthetic products, as I believe these life-sustaining nutrients should be obtained directly from nature through plant-based whole foods. I am, however, realistic about the fact that in our busy, highly industrialized society, accomplishing this noble task can be difficult.

As a busy working mom of three, I do rely on Juice Plus+®—a healthy, natural, whole food -and plant-based supplement—to boost my family's nutritional intake. I would like to highlight the fact that Juice Plus+® has a nutrition fact label rather than a supplement label, indicating that it is indeed just food.

In general, I tend to advise my patients to exercise caution whenever they take supplements with a supplement fact label, as this industry is not regulated by the Food and Drug Administration, and to steer toward products that bear the nutrition facts label. For more information on Juice Plus+®, please refer to www.drcynthia.com/juiceplus.

Numerous clinical studies in peer-reviewed scientific journals have shown that Juice Plus+® provides those who drink it with valuable phytonutrients and antioxidants, reduces oxidative stress, reduces biomarkers of inflammation, decreases homocysteine levels, and strengthens the immune system.

Research by the University of Maryland School of Medicine showed improved vascular compliance of the brachial artery and increased blood flow after a single high-fat meal after taking Juice Plus+®. A pilot study from Vanderbilt University School of Medicine likewise suggested improved vascular compliance from Juice Plus+®, and furthermore demonstrated a slowing of coronary artery calcification, raising interest for further vascular studies related to this supplement.

MINERALS

Minerals are inorganic elements needed by the body in small amounts for structure and to regulate chemical reactions in the body. In today's diet, minerals come from both plant and animal sources and are found in foods from all food groups.

Calcium

Calcium is the most abundant mineral in the body. Many people already know that calcium is important for healthy bones and teeth. However, calcium is also essential for a healthy heart and for cellular function. This mineral helps to conduct electricity in the heart, strengthens the blood vessels, prevents blood clotting, and staves off hypertension.

Calcium can be found in green vegetables such as broccoli, spinach, and collard greens, as well as in seaweed, hazelnuts, almonds, and rhubarb. Dairy products are also high in calcium, although in general people should avoid dairy products and look to soy milk, almond milk, or orange juice that has been fortified with calcium instead.

It should be noted that foods high in sugar and caffeine can inhibit the absorption of calcium in the body. Moreover, the elderly need extra calcium to counterbalance excess stomach acid, which can also prevent the body from absorbing calcium.

Copper

A lack of copper in the body can lead to elevated cholesterol levels, blood clotting, and heart disease. Copper contains essential enzymes that the arteries need to maintain their elasticity. In addition, copper has antioxidant properties that prevent inflammation and cell damage.

A study at the University of Louisville Medical Center suggests that copper may also be beneficial for people who have heart disease. In the study, two groups of mice with cardiac hypertrophy were fed diets containing various levels of copper. Cardiac hypertrophy is when the heart becomes enlarged after heart disease or high blood pressure. After four weeks, the hearts of the mice that ate high levels of copper returned to normal size, while the hearts of mice that ate low levels of copper did not.

You can find copper in nuts such as peanuts, macadamia nuts, and chestnuts, as well as leafy greens, chocolate, and oysters.

Magnesium

Magnesium is a mineral that affects the metabolism of calcium, sodium, and potassium in the human body. Magnesium may just be the most important mineral we need to prevent heart disease, diabetes, and stroke. The reason for this is because magnesium acts as a muscle relaxant, which eases tension of the arteries caused by high blood pressure. This muscle relaxation also helps to regulate your heartbeat so that oxygen-rich blood can be pumped efficiently to your vital organs and muscles.

Magnesium also controls blood sugar levels, reduces homocysteine levels, and prevents bone loss. Studies show that people who have low magnesium levels often suffer fatigue, muscle spasms, abnormal heart rhythms, seizures, vomiting, and insomnia. Researchers at the Duke University Medical Center found that people who had low magnesium levels were twice as likely to suffer heart attacks than people who had healthy levels of magnesium.

Experts suggest we should consume 500 to 700 milligrams of magnesium a day to ward off heart disease and diabetes. Some foods that are high in magnesium include spinach, whole grains, avocados, squash, soybeans, cashews, and almonds.

Potassium, Sodium, and Chloride

The water in our bodies contains a variety of mineral salts that are needed in proper amounts and combinations to maintain life. The minerals potassium, chloride, and sodium are the principal electrolytes in body fluids. Almost all of the sodium, chloride, and potassium consumed in the diet are absorbed.

The modern American diet is high in salt (sodium chloride) and low in potassium. The reason for this is primarily because we consume mostly processed foods—which are high in sodium—and not enough fresh unprocessed foods such as fruits and vegetables, which are low in sodium and high in potassium.

One of the biggest benefits of potassium is that it compensates for high sodium levels. The AHA suggests 4,700 milligrams of potassium a day for healthy heart function. An excess of sodium can cause fluid retention, which exerts pressure on the arteries. Potassium works to dismiss fluid retention and helps the muscles to contract for healthy cardiovascular function. Potassium also regulates heart rhythm and lowers blood pressure.

Studies show that people who follow the Dietary Approaches to Stop Hypertension (DASH) diet experience significant decreases in blood pressure and lower cholesterol levels. The DASH diet emphasis a variety of fruits and vegetables and includes low-fat dairy products. The foods allowed on the DASH eating plan are high in potassium, magnesium, fiber, and calcium, and low in saturated fats and sodium. You can find potassium in bananas, potatoes, broccoli, and winter squashes.

Zinc

Studies show that zinc can reduce inflammation in the body. Zinc is important because inflammation is a huge risk factor for cardiovascular disease. In addition, zinc can help lower levels of C-reactive protein and clear out old cholesterol building up in the arteries, which makes zinc an essential mineral for anyone suffering from atherosclerosis. You can find zinc in nuts, beans, and oysters.

DIETARY RECOMMENDATIONS FOR A HEALTHY HEART

The following are some dietary recommendations to keep your heart healthy and strong.

HEALTHY FATS: ESSENTIAL FATTY ACIDS

Essential fatty acids are necessary fats that humans cannot synthesize and therefore must be consumed through diet. Essential fatty acids (EFAs) help our cardiovascular, nervous, reproductive, and immune systems to function the way they are supposed to, and can protect us from diseases. With obesity and excess weight on the rise, we are constantly told by doctors, nutritionists, and the media that fat is bad. However, we actually need some "good fats" in our diet so that our body can perform basic functions.

Omega-3

Our bodies need essential fatty acids for proper vision, brain power, and healthy heart function. Omega-3 fatty acids contain docosahexaenoic acid (DHA) and eicosapentaenoic acid (EPA), which have been proven to lower blood pressure, stimulate circulation, decrease triglyceride levels, and increase the level of HDL, or good cholesterol, in the body. In addition, omega-3 fatty acids may prevent blood clotting by inhibiting the production of a chemical called thromboxane A2 and a protein called fibrin, both of which cause platelets in the blood to stick together.

Our bodies do not naturally synthesize omega-3, so we must get this vital nutrient from the foods we eat. The best sources of omega-3 fatty acids are cold-water fish such as salmon, sardines, tuna, and mackerel. According to the University of Maryland Medical Center, just two servings of fish every week can reduce your risk of stroke by 50 percent.

However, the problem is that certain types of fish can have very high fat content. In addition, as discussed earlier, there are health issues related to environmental toxins, both in wild-caught and farm-raised fish. The better options for obtaining omega-3 are soybeans, walnuts, chia seeds, pumpkin seeds, and flaxseeds.

Omega-6

Omega-6 (linoleic acid) is another essential fatty acid that contributes to healthy growth, proper metabolism, and bodily functions. The body converts linoleic acid to gamma-linolenic acid (GLA), which works with omega-3 to help fight inflammation, lower blood pressure, and prevent blood clotting. Omega-6 can be found in plant oils such as sunflower oil, flaxseed oil, olive oil, and blackcurrant oil. It can also be found in pistachios, eggs, sunflower seeds, and pumpkin seeds.

It is important to note that too much omega-6 can be a bad thing. High levels of omega-6 that are not counterbalanced with equal or more levels of omega-3 in the body can cause inflammation. Therefore, it is important to have a healthy balance of both omega-3 and omega-6.

PROTEIN

Protein is essential for life, as it contributes to healthy muscles and joints, cellular processes, and proper blood flow. This macronutrient also balances the pH level of the blood by adding and removing hydrogen ions when needed. It furthermore facilitates in transporting nutrients throughout the body and removing toxins from the bloodstream.

Protein can be found in meat, vegetables, nuts, seeds, and legumes. When it comes to heart-healthy protein intake, the Harvard School of Public Health suggests replacing red meat with poultry, fish, nuts, and beans to lower your risk of heart disease, diabetes, and premature death as a result of cardiovascular disease.

COMPLEX CARBOHYDRATES

You may have heard that carbohydrates can lead to weight gain. This is certainly true, although it depends on the type of carbs you consume. Simple carbohydrates are converted into glucose in the body soon after they are consumed. This means that your blood sugar levels soar for a short period before crashing again. In addition, the body stores simple carbs as fat, which can lead to weight gain.

On the other hand, complex carbohydrates are broken down gradually by the body, so the glucose is slowly released into your bloodstream and used for energy. In this way, complex carbs help to control blood sugar and insulin levels, which is good for people with type 2 diabetes. In addition, these types of carbs can help lower cholesterol and blood pressure.

Dietary fiber is included in complex carbohydrates and is absolutely essential for detoxification and heart health. According to the AHA, studies show that foods high in fiber can prevent heart disease. One way that fiber reduces the risk of cardiovascular disease is by binding to LDL cholesterol in the intestines so that the cholesterol cannot be absorbed by the body. This prevents clogged arteries.

In addition, fiber helps to flush toxins from the body through the intestines. This prevents free-radical damage and promotes a healthy circulatory system. Moreover, fiber regulates blood sugar and insulin levels.

Complex carbohydrates and dietary fiber can be found in whole grains such as rye, oats, brown rice, and whole wheat, as well as in fruits and vegetables such as broccoli, mushrooms, bell peppers, onions, beans, cauliflower, kale, grapefruits, and oranges. It is important to eat whole foods rather than refined or processed foods, as the latter often contain simple carbohydrates that are bad for the body.

DAILY RECOMMENDATIONS

Eating a balanced diet of wholesome foods is critical to maintaining healthy body chemistry. The AHA suggests eating 4.5 cups of fruits and vegetables a day, three servings of whole grains a day, four servings of nuts, seeds, and legumes a week, and two servings of fish a week. In addition, it recommends lowering your sodium intake to 1,500 milligrams or less a day, and eating processed meats no more than twice a week.

My personal belief is to avoid all animal protein and dairy products, or else to minimize the intake by starting with one or two servings of fish weekly and then building your oral intake around plant-based whole foods from there. Initially, considering a healthful diet omitting all animal products, including fish, sounds daunting.

Here is a simple way to get there: try plant-based foods for one to two weeks to appreciate the variety of options and see which foods you might like. When you are ready, try 100 percent plant-based foods for three weeks; see how you do and, more importantly, how you feel. Let your body be the judge, but only after you have given your body and mind a fair chance to appreciate the difference they would feel with a plant-based diet.

The well-recognized USDA food pyramid published by the World Health Organization (WHO) and the Food and Agriculture Organization

(FAO) in 1992 contained bread, cereal, rice, and pasta as the broad base and allowed for whole-milk and animal-protein intake.

The latest effort by the USDA to restructure nutritional guidelines led to the MyPlate program in 2011, depicting four quadrants comprising vegetables, fruits, grains, and protein. While this program is more reflective of the latest dietetic research, it still is an oversimplification and is vague in the recommendations.

I prefer Dr. Fuhrman's Nutritarian Food Pyramid, as it more accurately depicts an increased consumption of highly dense, nutrient-rich, plant-based foods and a decreased intake of low-nutrient, high-calorie foods. In addition, the Nutritarian Food Plate specifies the sources of healthy fat, protein, and whole grains.

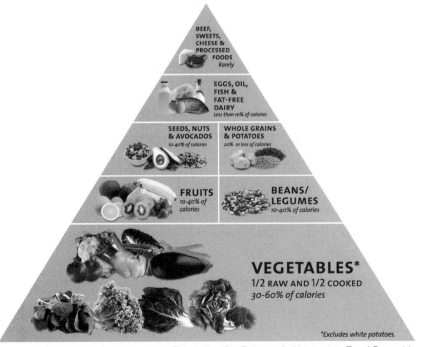

Fig. 3-3   Dr. Fuhrman's Nutritarian Food Pyramid

B R A N C H I N G   O U T

Nutrition is only beginning to gain a firm foothold in the medical community. Dr. Neal Barnard and the Physicians Committee for Responsible Medicine (www.pcrm.org), of which I am a member, are making a critical outreach to the next generation of physicians by providing the Nutrition Guide for Clinicians, cowritten by Barnard, to second-year medical students. It is vitally important that comprehensive nutritional education be at the forefront of training for new physicians.

I urge my patients and readers to become more knowledgeable about nutrition, the various food sources, and their effects on the body. A documentary that I highly recommend is *Forks Over Knives*, which had a profound effect on me and greatly expanded my own knowledge base on this subject. It presents a very compelling argument against the consumption of animal protein and dairy.

The film chronicles the journeys of two researchers, Dr. T. Colin Campbell, a nutritional scientist at Cornell University (coauthor of *The China Study*), and Dr. Caldwell Esselstyn, a leading surgeon at the Cleveland Clinic (heart-disease reversal study), in their independent discoveries that many of the chronic degenerative diseases, such as heart disease, diabetes, and several forms of cancer, are virtually nonexistent in areas of the world where there is little or no consumption of animal-based food.

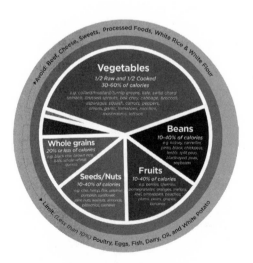

Fig. 3-4   Dr. Fuhrman's Nutritarian Food Plate

Another documentary worth viewing is *Fat, Sick & Nearly Dead*, featuring the self-healing journey of an Australian man called Joe Cross. Cross was diagnosed with a debilitating autoimmune condition, weighed over 300 pounds, and was on multiple medications. The film shows him traveling through America, the land of his greatest temptations, documenting his sixty-day fruit- and vegetable-juicing fast to reclaim his health.

Also featured in this documentary is Phil Staples—a morbidly obese truck driver from Iowa, who weighed 429 pounds and suffered from the same rare condition—who reached out and asked for help to transform his life. What emerges is a truly inspirational, uplifting story of two remarkable men on personal self-healing, life-reclaiming journeys.

Cross and Staples demonstrate the power of a purposeful vision, deliberate action, and free will to achieve what all the medical technology, pharmaceutical drugs, and physicians cannot: freedom from life-threatening immunologic disease and the achievement of optimal health and a vibrant heart!

If we are to significantly impact our health, it is vitally important that we educate ourselves and our children on this vast topic of nutrition and our food supply. Two visionaries—the father-and-son team of John and Ocean Robbins—have made this concept possible and practical by providing a comprehensive discussion of these topics through their Food Revolution Network (www.yourvibrantheart.com/foodrev). As revolutionary as its name suggests, the network is spearheading the effort to change the way we think about our food and its production.

The latest in research on the topic is provided by twenty-four of the world's top experts in the movement for promoting healthy, sustainable, humane, and conscious food, all of them sharing their insights on the links between diet, health, and the future of our food in their annual Food Revolution Summit.

THE LINK BETWEEN FOOD AND ENERGY

The effects of healthy foods extend far beyond the physical. Bad nutrition leads to an increase in the insulin circulating through our blood, which in turn causes brain fog. This fog prevents us from being focused and connecting with our inner guides. Moreover, eating bad foods means that the body needs to expend more energy detoxing itself—energy that it could be using to achieve spiritual clarity. Feeding your body well is therefore the preliminary step in achieving a strong mental and spiritual connection in your life.

It doesn't stop there. Food itself is energy. When we cook or microwave food, we destroy more than just the nutrients and the enzymes that it contains. We are destroying life itself. Therefore, when we eat whole foods, we are absorbing the pure energy that we are meant to be nourished with, and we are nurturing ourselves on a much deeper level than we are when we consume dead foods. In these ways, nutrition is fundamentally linked not only with our physical health, but with our mental and spiritual health as well.

CHAPTER 4

FITNESS FOR YOUR HEART

*"You live longer once you realize that any time spent being unhappy
is wasted."*

—Ruth E. Renkl

People who exercise on a regular basis are not only healthier than those
who don't, but they are also happier and more relaxed, and have more
energy. The health benefits of exercise are huge, as regular aerobic and
strength-training sessions can help reduce high blood pressure and bad
cholesterol in the body. This in turn can prevent heart attacks, strokes, and
other cardiac conditions.

Your heart is a muscle, and like any muscle, it needs exercise to keep
strong and healthy. Contrary to popular belief, exercise does not have to be
strenuous, boring, or expensive. There are many ways you can incorporate
exercise into your lifestyle in an enjoyable
and inexpensive manner.

Many people underestimate the way
that physical exercise can contribute to
your mental and physical awareness. Exercising can calm the mind and put you into

Exercising
can calm the
mind and put
you into an almost
meditative state.

an almost meditative state. In the Western world, we refer to this as being "in the zone."

Stanford researcher Dr. Bruce Lipton has postulated that we are controlled 5 percent by our conscious mind and 95 percent by our subconscious mind. When we are engaged in an activity such as driving a car, that is our subconscious mind at work. The same is true of exercise.

When you play sports or engage in a physical activity, your positive subconscious takes over. If you try to think too hard on a basketball court about what your posture is like and how your hand should be and who is coming up to guard you, you're going to miss all of the shots. On the other hand, if you enter "the zone" and allow your subconscious to take over your actions, you play well.

This state of being physically present without being consciously present is a form of meditation. Your mind empties itself of the clutter that normally crowds it, and you achieve clarity. This then connects back to your physical health when you consider that, during meditation, all kinds of bad stress and adrenaline hormones in the body settle down. Meditation combats things like cortisol, a steroid hormone, and thus can help with illnesses such as heart disease and diabetes. Here we can see the physiology of a spiritual act.

There are many forms of exercise that you can do to strengthen the heart, tone the muscles, burn fat, and feel healthier, happier, and more confident. The best exercises for the heart are cardiovascular or aerobic exercises. These could include activities like walking, running, cycling, or swimming. Strength training can also have very positive effects on your cardiovascular health by lowering your blood pressure and building muscle to reduce strain on your heart.

Finally, Eastern practices such as yoga and tai chi can reduce stress, lower blood pressure and cholesterol, strengthen your core, improve blood circulation, and promote healthy breathing practices. The best way to start is to choose a few exercises that you enjoy, and slowly introduce them into your schedule.

For optimum heart health, you should do twenty to thirty minutes of aerobic exercise a day, three to four times a week. For strength training, you should add two or three sessions of thirty minutes each into your schedule per week.

Every workout should begin with a warm-up that includes gentle stretches to loosen up your muscles and prevent injury and strain. This should be followed by your cardio or strength-training workout. After the workout session, you should spend about five to ten minutes cooling down with some stretches and low-intensity movements.

THE BENEFITS OF STRETCHING

The most common mistake people make when starting a workout session is to neglect to stretch before and after their exercise session. Stretching is the key to avoiding painful injuries. Your body needs time to limber up, get the blood flowing, and slowly ease into a state of deeper breathing and increased heart rate. This is also true at the end of the workout, as your body needs time to ease back into a state of rest.

The important thing to remember with stretching is to keep it simple. Ease into the stretches slowly and gently, and try not to make sudden movements or bounce while in position. Hold the stretch for a few seconds, and then slowly ease out. If you feel pain at any point, gently pull out of the stretch and move on to something different.

Each stretch should be repeated two or three times to loosen up the muscles. A good warm-up and cool-down session should last about five to ten minutes, and it should target many different muscle groups.

LEARNING TO STRETCH

Stretching may seem like a simple exercise that does nothing to build muscle or work out your heart. However, neglecting to stretch before a bout of physical activity can lead to serious injuries.

One of my patients had a daughter named Kyra who was a snowboarding instructor. Kyra would take groups of small children up the mountain to practice their turns daily. Throughout her shift she was constantly moving, riding down the slopes, helping the kids to get up when they fell, and twisting and turning to keep an eye on her students.

Kyra never thought to stretch before her shift, as she was young, full of energy, and never had problems. That is, until one day when Kyra woke up with intense pain in her neck and down through her right shoulder. It was so severe that she could barely turn her head. She missed three days of work because she could not move properly, which was essential for her job.

A trip to the chiropractor revealed that her injury was due to a lack of stretching. Now, Krya stretches before every shift, and the problem has not returned.

CARDIOVASCULAR OR AEROBIC EXERCISE

Cardiovascular or aerobic exercise is any form of physical activity that gets your heart beating faster and your lungs expanding and breathing deeper. Good cardiovascular health is vital for a long and healthy life.

One reason aerobic exercise is good for your heart is that it causes your heart to expand. When your heart expands, it increases its stroke volume (amount of blood pumped with each heartbeat) and takes in more oxygen. This allows your body to use the oxygen in a more efficient way, which lowers blood pressure. In addition, aerobic exercise can lower your resting heart rate.

Medical experts agree that a resting heart rate under sixty beats per minute is a sign of a healthy heart. The longer it takes for your heart rate to go above one hundred during a vigorous workout and the quicker it comes down below one hundred after finishing the workout reflect the physical condition of your heart.

The level of physical fitness and the activities and strenuous level of those activities necessary to achieve optimal conditioning varies from individual to individual.

I always remind my patients that there is never a bar on physical fitness … you can never reach the pinnacle of endurance . . . there is always a higher benchmark to target. I encourage people to always build improvement into their workout; in other words, never be satisfied with the level of fitness you have achieved and work toward achieving just that much more. Whether you are Kevin Durant, David Beckham, or an eighty-year-old grandmother, you have your own standards and bars to improve upon.

According to the CDC, regular aerobic activity can lower your risk of heart disease and stroke, decrease your chances of developing type 2 diabetes and certain cancers, lower blood pressure and LDL (bad) cholesterol while increasing HDL (good) cholesterol, control weight, strengthen bones and muscles, improve your mental health and mood, and allow you to live longer. The CDC recommends doing about 150 minutes of aerobic exercise a week, spread out over seven days.

Incorporating cardiovascular exercise into your life is easy because there are so many forms of exercise to choose from. You can try walking, jogging, swimming, cycling, skipping rope, or even working out at home with your Wii.

The best part is that many of these cardiovascular exercises require nothing more than a decent pair of shoes. You do not need a pricey gym membership or fancy exercise equipment to enjoy a good aerobic workout. To make the workouts more fun, grab a friend or a pet, and get outside and enjoy the fresh air while strengthening your heart and toning your body at the same time. After just a few weeks you will feel more relaxed, healthy, and joyful.

WALKING

Walking is one of the most natural forms of aerobic exercise you can do. This is a great form of exercise for beginners because it is very low impact and low intensity, and therefore it does not cause a great deal of strain on the body. Moreover, walking has a great deal of positive health benefits. It can:

- Lower LDL (bad) cholesterol

- Raise HDL (good) cholesterol

- Lower high blood pressure

- Prevent or manage type 2 diabetes

- Burn fat and maintain a healthy body weight

- Fight depression and anxiety

- Strengthen muscles and bones and tone the body

RUNNING OR JOGGING

Running is another natural form of exercise that is more challenging than walking, with increased health benefits from a more vigorous exercise regimen. Although moderate activity is beneficial to the heart and body, more benefits can be obtained from higher-intensity workouts like running.

Running gets the heart pumping blood and oxygen more efficiently. The amount of blood your heart delivers to the body is called cardiac output (liters/minute) or stroke volume (ml/heartbeat) and can have a tremendous impact on your energy level and endurance. The typical cardiac output is four to six liters with a stroke volume of sixty to eighty ml/heartbeat, but the values can range as low as less than two liters a minute to higher than ten liters a minute in an athlete.

A study by the American College of Sports Medicine (ACSM) revealed that people who ran fifty miles a week or more showed a dramatic decrease in body fat and triglyceride levels, as well as an increase in good HDL cholesterol, when compared to people who only ran ten miles a week. In addition, the people who ran fifty miles a week managed to reduce their blood pressure by 50 percent. Running encourages the heart and peripheral muscles to work better, burns calories, and is one of the best forms of exercise to lose weight.

SWIMMING

Swimming is an excellent form of cardiovascular exercise because it works out the entire body. It is also a very low-impact form of exercise, so it is gentle on the joints. Even people with injuries or stiff joints can benefit from a swimming workout. A vigorous swimming session works out more muscles than any other form of exercise, so it is a great way to get a lean, toned body. Moreover, swimming increases your respiratory and heart rates, which improves your cardiovascular and lung function.

I recently had a visit from Robert with his ten-year-old daughter. Since our last visit, he had lost ten pounds and he looked healthier and more energized. I knew that physical activity and exercise had always been a roadblock for him. In our previous discussion, he had said he felt that exercise was a chore to be avoided like the plague.

When I inquired about his activities, he said he had started going to the beach with his daughter and that he had gotten reintroduced to his love of surfing. He now spends hours on the weekend fighting the waves, and without knowing it, he had slowly improved his endurance. Summer was over, but with renewed enthusiasm over his improvement, he started going swimming.

CYCLING

Cycling is another form of low-impact aerobic exercise that is great for losing weight and developing a strong heart and respiratory system. Oxygen is vital for your body to function, and sedentary people often suffer from poor respiration.

Regular moderate physical activity like cycling can strengthen the muscles used in your respiratory system, which allows the lungs to take in more oxygen. In addition, cycling gives the heart a good workout, which reduces stress on this vital organ. This helps to reduce the risk of heart attacks. Moreover, cycling encourages the body to use up fat reserves. Maintaining a healthy weight prevents damage to your vital organs.

According to the British Medical Association, people who cycle up to twenty miles a week can reduce their risk of coronary disease by up to 50 percent. In addition, cycling lowers your blood pressure and regulates cholesterol levels, favoring beneficial cholesterol over the harmful type. This can decrease your risk of strokes and heart disease.

Use a bicycle as a means of transportation to save money, decrease your carbon footprint, and stay fit. You can also jump on the stationary bike at the gym to keep track of your heart rate and the amount of calories you burn each session. This is a great way to reduce stress, burn fat, and feed the soul.

SKIPPING

There is a reason why many top athletes start their workouts with a skipping session. Skipping gets the heart beating faster, encourages the lungs to work at full capacity, and burns twice as many calories as a brisk walking session. Jumping rope is also an effective way to build muscle and bone density. The Osteoporosis Society of the United Kingdom recommends skipping every day for two to five minutes to ward off osteoporosis. This inexpensive and portable form of exercise can improve your balance, coordination, flexibility, and agility.

ROWING

Rowing is a total-body workout that burns calories, improves respiratory function, and gets the blood flowing for optimum heart health. This type of aerobic exercise requires your lungs to take in a great deal of oxygen, which strengthens your respiratory muscles such as the diaphragm, and expands the alveoli, or the air sacs in your lungs. This allows your lungs to develop an increased ability to process oxygen.

By adopting regular rowing workouts, you can also strengthen your heart. According to the ACSM, a stronger and healthier heart will make you less prone to disease and illness. Rowing can also improve the condition of your blood vessels by preventing blockages, and increasing elasticity. This contributes to healthy blood pressure levels.

HIGH-INTENSITY INTERVAL TRAINING

While cardiovascular exercise has many obvious benefits, there is evidence to suggest that excessive cardio may be counterproductive and potentially even harmful. A Canadian study revealed that sustained vigorous exercise can actually increase your cardiac risk. Another study published by the *European Heart Journal* showed that exercise induced right-ventricular dysfunction and increased blood levels of cardiac enzymes, signifying cellular damage. The journal also provided evidence for the development of scar tissues in the heart muscles of athletes after endurance races.

There is now a growing body of evidence that high-intensity interval training is a more effective and efficient way to develop cardiovascular benefits. If one looks at the evolution of our ancestors, the hunter-gatherers used bursts of physical activity, followed by substantial periods of rest, to function on a day-to-day basis. Our bodies are not designed for sustained bouts of physical activity, and when this activity occurs—such as in a marathon—the body produces stress hormones and develops enzymes that enable it to store fat.

By contrast, interval training involves bursts of maximum cardiovascular activity, sustained for only thirty-second to one-minute intervals, followed by slower-paced recovery periods of ninety seconds to three minutes. This cycle is then repeated six to eight times to complete the workout. The benefits of interval training include improved exercise capacity, better metabolism, higher insulin resistance, healthier blood pressure, stronger HDL levels, and reduced body fat.

TEAM SPORTS

Team sports are a great way to improve your physical and mental health, and get some social interaction at the same time. According to the United Nations Inter-Agency Task Force on Sport for Development and Peace, sports help young people develop strong bones and healthy hearts and lungs, and improve their coordination and motor skills. Adults can also benefit from sports, which help to improve heart health and overall movement.

Team sports such as basketball, soccer, and volleyball can get your heart rate up and your endorphins pumping. They can also build muscles and improve heart and lung strength. All of these elements combine to improve your cardiovascular health, lower your risk for common colds and disease, prevent injuries and pain, and battle depression by producing a natural euphoria. Moreover, you will lose weight and tone your body, which will help with self-confidence and body awareness.

Cardiovascular exercise is vital to optimum health. However, it is important to note that people who are at a high risk for cardiovascular conditions, or those who suffer from weak joints, are recovering from injuries, or are taking medications, should consult with their doctor before starting an aerobic exercise program.

MIND-BODY AXIS

TEAM SPIRIT

Beyond being physically good for you, the camaraderie and cooperation built into team sports work to strengthen your mental resolve in addition to your physical strength. The social aspect of team sports can improve your communication skills and lower social anxiety. In contrast to individual sports, team sports give you the feeling of being a piece of the pie and a part of the puzzle. You receive validation not only from yourself, but also from your coaches, teammates, and supporters. This aspect of team activity takes sports beyond the physical benefits to your heart and muscles. It strengthens your mind and spirit, too.

STRENGTH TRAINING

Strength training, or resistance training, builds muscle and burns fat, resulting in a leaner, more toned body. Strength training is also good for cardiovascular health.

In 2000, the AHA published a report in *Circulation: Journal of the American Heart Association*, stating that resistance training could greatly benefit heart health for people in good health. The report confirmed that strength training not only increases muscle strength and endurance, but that it also improves cardiovascular function and reduces the risk of coronary disease. The AHA later expanded on this study, reporting in 2007 that resistance training could benefit people who are recovering from heart disease.

Resistance training works out the muscles and the cardiovascular system at the same time. Strength training involves using weights, resistance machines or bands, or your own body to contract the muscles and resist against weight. This increases your strength and endurance by building your muscles and bone density, and by getting the blood circulating.

Moderate weight training can increase the heart rate, which helps to improve heart function. In addition, the stronger the muscles are, the less stress there is on the blood vessels, lungs, and heart. This helps to protect your vital organs and to keep your heart healthy and strong. Strength training also lowers your bad LDL cholesterol and blood pressure, and boosts metabolism. Moreover, studies by the AHA show that resistance exercises can also reduce the symptoms of other health conditions such as arthritis, osteoporosis, lower back pain, obesity, and diabetes.

The AHA suggests that people add two to three strength-training sessions to their fitness plan every week to significantly decrease their chances of heart disease. Each training session should include ten to twelve repetitions of eight to ten discrete exercises, with a minimum of one exercise per major muscle group twice a week to complement your cardio workout.

Examples of exercises that target major muscle groups include a chest press, shoulder press, triceps extension, biceps curl, pull-down (upper back), lower-back extension, abdominal crunch/curl-up, quadriceps extension or leg press, leg curls (hamstrings), and calf raise.

Now more than ever, medical experts call for strength-training programs to improve cardiovascular health, prevent and alleviate symptoms of disease, and boost physical and mental health. If done properly, strength training can also increase your strength and stamina, boost insulin metabolism, help you lose weight and sleep deeper, and improve your overall mood. As opposed to aerobic exercise, which does not appear

TIPS FOR SAFE STRENGTH-TRAINING EXERCISES

- *Before lifting weights or doing resistance training, warm up with a few minutes of light cardio activity. After the resistance training, do some gentle stretches to cool down. This will help to prevent injuries, aches, and pains.*
- *Start off slowly with a weight that you are comfortable with. Once you have built up your resistance, you can gradually add more weight.*
- *Use slow, controlled movements to follow through the full range of motion for each muscle group you work on.*
- *Use high-intensity, super-slow strength training to gain maximum benefit in a shorter period of time.*
- *Breathe out when you are contracting your muscles, and inhale when you are at a state of rest.*
- *Do not hold your breath while doing the exercises.*
- *If you are working out with large or heavy weights such as barbells, have someone spot you in case you need help lifting the weights out of position.*
- *Try to repeat each strength-training exercise eight to ten times to see the best results.*

to have a sustained fat burn after exercise, strength training leads to a prolonged increase in metabolism and a continued fat burn after exercise.

Building strength in your upper body helps to support your heart and lungs by putting less strain on them. In this way, these organs can do their job better and pump more oxygen throughout the body using fewer heartbeats.

Strength training is an excellent way to prevent disease and helps to rehabilitate the heart after a coronary episode. In addition, by making your body stronger and increasing your endurance, you make it easier to do simple everyday tasks like walking up stairs or lifting heavy objects.

It is important to note that strength training is best suited to people who are at a low risk for cardiac conditions. The AHA suggests that people do not lift weights if they have the following heart conditions:

- Unstable coronary heart disease, such as angina
- Congestive heart failure
- Severe pulmonary hypertension
- Severe, symptomatic aortic stenosis
- Acute infection of the heart or tissues surrounding the heart
- Uncontrolled high blood pressure that is greater than 180/110 mmHg
- Aortic dissection
- Marfan syndrome

If you suspect that you may have a heart condition, speak to your doctor before embarking on a strength-training program.

EASTERN PRACTICES

Many Eastern cultures have a long history of holistic practices that aim to connect the body and mind, reduce stress and tension, improve overall health, and prevent disease.

Many of these practices focus on slow, controlled movements, mindful breathing techniques, and allowing energy to flow freely through the body. This is extremely beneficial for building muscle and bone density, improving blood circulation, and lowering blood pressure. Studies show that people who do yoga, tai chi, martial arts, or qigong on a regular basis can significantly lower their risk of heart disease and stroke, as well as many other illnesses.

Although many of these traditional Eastern exercises may not increase the heart rate to the same extent as other forms of physical activity, they do have a dramatic effect with dilating the blood vessels and improving blood flow. Holding the postures that many of these exercises entail strengthens the body's core in a way that many Western-style forms of exercise fail to do.

For instance, my husband spends an hour a day at the gym. He runs half an hour on the treadmill and does strength training with the other half. One day, he came to yoga with me. Neither of us thought that it would be all that difficult for him, but he couldn't keep up. He just couldn't hold the postures for two to three minutes—his abdominal core wasn't strong enough.

There are many professional athletes who have discovered that yoga and other forms of Eastern exercises provide them with a different form of real physical training that they don't get from their standard routines.

Many Eastern cultures have a long history of holistic practices that aim to connect the body and mind, reduce stress and tension, improve overall health, and prevent disease.

YOGA

Yoga is an ancient Indian practice that has become very popular the world over for its ability to ward off certain illnesses, reduce stress, and tone the body. According to the Harvard Medical School, yoga may lower the risk factors related to cardiovascular failure, including high cholesterol levels, blood sugars, and blood pressure. Moreover, yoga may encourage the heart to recover and heal from a cardiac episode, improve respiratory function, and ease heart palpitations and the symptoms of heart failure and arthritis.

Yoga also promotes a lifestyle that is very beneficial to heart health. The practice encourages relaxation, reduces stress and negativity, and allows the body to perform necessary functions with ease.

Coronary heart disease and the factors that contribute to cardiovascular failure can be brought on by inactivity, stress, and a poor diet. Yoga can combat these risk factors by combining exercise, meditation, and a better self-awareness of bodily functions. In addition, yoga can slow the aging process by detoxifying the body.

STAYING YOUNG WITH YOGA

Edward was a patient of mine who had a very active lifestyle, but not necessarily in a healthy sense. Although he was in his forties, he was unmarried, had no children, and enjoyed going out dancing and socializing with his friends most nights of the week.

Eventually, Edward got tired of the party lifestyle and decided to explore other ways of expending his energy. He took a yoga course and liked it so much that he decided to enroll in a Bikram Yoga teacher training course in Los Angeles. Edward went on to travel to India to see the birthplace of yoga and eventually accepted a job teaching in Bangkok, Thailand.

I had not seen Edward for a number of years, but one day I got a call from him saying he was in Burbank for a few days. He made an appointment to see me.

When I walked into the exam room, I was in total shock! He looked like a completely different person. He was much slimmer with lean muscles. In addition, he looked about ten years younger. His skin was clear, his eyes were bright, his posture was straight and tall, and he had a healthy vigor about him. I mentioned this to him, and he said, "You would not believe how many people say that to me. I guess that's what yoga does for you."

Yoga for Heart Health and Diabetes

Practitioners of yoga can prevent and control heart disease and diabetes to a certain extent. Studies have shown that Kapalabhati, a controlled breathing technique used in many yoga practices, can lower blood glucose levels and increase the amount of oxygen that is absorbed into the blood stream. This helps the heart function better and strengthens the respiratory system.

In addition, the meditative aspect of yoga reduces stress, which brings the heart rate down and lowers blood pressure. Furthermore, the movements in yoga improve circulation through better elasticity of the arteries, lower cholesterol, and decrease the risk of heart disease, strokes, and diabetes.

Hatha yoga is an excellent form of relaxing, meditative yoga that brings down stress levels and eases tension. The sun salutations used in this practice are good for getting the blood circulating and regulating the heart rhythm. Ashtanga yoga is a more vigorous form of yoga that can be compared to an aerobic workout. It focuses on building strength and endurance, and it includes controlled breathing exercises. This is great for people who want a more energetic workout. People with heart problems and high blood pressure should generally avoid Bikram or Hot Yoga, which is practiced in rooms heated to 105 degrees Fahrenheit and can be a very intense experience.

Dahn yoga is the particular form of yoga that my family and I practice. Its founder, Ilchi Lee, author of *The Call of Sedona*, developed this training program based on ancient Korean practices. His book served as my guide on my recent visit to that magnificent place, which I will describe later. I particularly appreciate this form of yoga because it incorporates and focuses on energy healing, especially as it relates to the brain and to our personal mindset.

Dahn yoga is a unique holistic energy-training program designed to teach people to work with their energy, especially when energy becomes stagnant in the body. As discussed earlier, stress energy can wreak havoc on our bodies, leading to high blood pressure, diabetes, depression, anxiety, and many other forms of dis "ease."

One exercise in Dahn yoga that is designed to help regulate stress energy is called Brain Wave Vibration (BWV). A study from the University of London and Korea Institute of Brain Science showed that BWV improved depression, stress, sleep latency, and mindfulness. I can say that this weekly practice has helped me to become more centered and has helped my children to become more focused.

The kind of yoga you choose to practice is up to your personal preference, experience, and fitness level. Regular practice of any type of this wonderful exercise can improve your balance, flexibility, energy levels, core strength, concentration, self-awareness, and overall mood. Furthermore, nearly every form of yoga includes postures that are designed to improve blood circulation and strengthen the heart.

MARTIAL ARTS

Contrary to popular belief, martial arts are not simply a form of self-defense or combat. Although many of the martial arts do contain an element of self-protection, they can also be used to improve heart health and minimize the risk of disease. In addition, they can tone the body, manage weight, and develop better balance, flexibility, and concentration.

Research by the *British Journal of Sports Medicine* concludes that adults in their forties and fifties who regularly practiced martial arts showed increased health benefits when compared to people who did not exercise. This included better agility, stronger immune systems, and up to 12 percent less body fat.

Additional studies show that martial arts can regulate blood sugar levels and stabilize the heart rate, which can decrease the risk of hypertension, type 2 diabetes, and coronary heart disease. In addition, the controlled movements and breathing in martial arts practices can reduce stress, depression, and fatigue.

TAI CHI

The ancient Chinese art of tai chi consists of a series of slow-moving exercises that can greatly improve heart health, concentration, and balance. The movements are based on the Chinese philosophy that each of us has a life force called qi (or chi) flowing through our bodies. Although its roots originate from a focus on martial arts, defense, and power, tai chi is increasingly used in modern times for health and spiritual purposes. The movements in tai chi are believed to get rid of blockages so that this life force can flow more freely throughout the body.

As the body shifts through the movements in tai chi, gentle pressure is exerted on the veins, which encourages blood to flow to the heart.

In addition, the deep-breathing techniques that are used in this practice allow oxygen to enter the blood cells. This detoxifies the body, balances blood sugar levels and hormones, and allows the blood vessels to expand, which can alleviate high blood pressure. In addition, the meditative aspect of tai chi can be very grounding, and many people find that they have less stress, anxiety, and depression after taking tai chi classes.

There have been many studies on the effects of tai chi on the body by prominent research centers such as the Harvard Medical School, the National Taiwan University, and Tufts University. These studies indicate that tai chi can alleviate the symptoms of arthritis, Parkinson's disease, hypertension, heart disease, and breast cancer. Patients in the studies who took tai chi for twelve weeks or more showed a dramatic decrease in bad LDL cholesterol, blood pressure, and triglycerides, as well as an improvement in flexibility, sleep patterns, breathing, and overall quality of life.

The movements in tai chi are very controlled, gentle, and grounding. In this way, they are perfect for people of all ages and fitness levels. Even

TAI CHI TIPS FOR BEGINNERS

If you are considering taking tai chi, here are some tips to get you started:

- Try sitting in on a class first to see if the practice is something you would be interested in. Many people find tai chi very relaxing and energizing, while others might prefer a more active and vigorous workout.

- Wear comfortable, loose-fitting clothing when practicing. This will allow you to breathe properly and move through the different positions with ease. Comfortable shoes are also a necessity, although some people practice in bare feet to feel more grounded.

- Try to stick to your tai chi program for at least twelve weeks. Most of the medical studies on tai chi show that the people who exhibited the most health benefits were the ones who had been practicing twice a week for about three months or more.

people with mobility problems can take tai chi without having to worry about injury or strain. This makes it an excellent form of exercise for people who suffer from heart problems or high blood pressure. Studies at the National Taiwan University revealed that people with a high risk for heart disease who took tai chi showed significant improvements in blood pressure, cholesterol, and C-reactive protein levels.

QIGONG

Another ancient Chinese practice, qigong, which dates back over four thousand years, has been known to produce very positive health benefits in practitioners. Like tai chi, qigong focuses on the life force or qi that flows throughout the body. Unlike tai chi, however, its roots are based predominantly in healing.

In a typical qigong session, practitioners concentrate on using slow, fluid movements and deep, mindful breathing techniques to encourage good blood flow, strong muscles, and better balance and flexibility. There is also an element of meditation in qigong, which aids in decreasing stress, tension, and depression.

Research shows that qigong can be very effective in lowering the heart rate, decreasing pain, and improving immune functions. In addition, the slow movements help to build muscle mass, which can aid in regulating blood pressure and strengthening the heart. Finally, studies show that regular qigong practice can also raise cortisol levels in the body. This is a hormone that the body produces to combat stress. Overall, there are many positive benefits to practicing qigong.

One of the best things about qigong is that anybody can do it. It is a very low-impact and low-intensity form of exercise, and it can be done standing, sitting, or even lying down. This means that even people who are recovering from surgery or injuries can practice qigong. Many people find that qigong can be very therapeutic, as it aims to integrate the mind, body, and spirit. Others see it as a form of prevention against disease as well as a healing and restorative practice. A free video training series from qigong master Lee Holden can be found on www. yourvibrantheart.com/qigong.

NIA

Created in 1983, NIA is a relatively new phenomenon in the world of fitness. NIA, which stands for neuromuscular integrative action, is a combination of slow and fast movements similar to those in tai chi, meditation, freestyle dance, and low-impact aerobic exercise.

In a typical NIA class, practitioners start off by listening to relaxing music, practicing deep-breathing exercises, meditating, and making slow movements to get the body warmed up. As the class progresses, the music changes to a more upbeat tempo, and students are encouraged to increase their range of motion, get the body moving, and increase their breathing. Students may be asked to visualize situations or make vocalizations as they shake and spin to release stress and create a better awareness of their bodies.

NIA can offer positive cardiovascular benefits to those who take classes on a regular basis. The controlled breathing exercises help to expand the lungs and allow more oxygen to be absorbed into the bloodstream. This helps the heart to pump blood throughout the body more efficiently. The full range of movements encourages better balance and flexibility, enhances blood circulation, and gets the heart rate up, which strengthens the cardiovascular system.

The classes also focus on reducing stress and anxiety, which are common causes of high blood pressure. Moreover, the classes can be adapted to people of all fitness levels, including cardiovascular patients who are in rehabilitation and stroke victims. This is an excellent way for people of all ages and fitness levels to get moving for optimal cardiovascular health.

People tend to think that risky behavior and poor lifestyle choices such as smoking, excessive alcohol consumption, and overeating are the main contributors to heart disease and poor health. While it is true that these factors greatly increase the risk of cardiac conditions, a sedentary lifestyle is just as bad. Living an active life is crucial to your health, vitality, and overall well-being.

By adding just a few sessions a week of cardio, strength training, and Eastern practices like yoga or qigong, you can decrease your risk of disease, increase your energy levels, and improve your mood. You will look and feel fitter, healthier, and more youthful. You will also nurture your mind and spirit by allowing your subconscious to take over for a while, giving you the opportunity to clear your mind and to enter a meditative state that supports health in every aspect of your being.

CHAPTER 5

REJUVENATE YOUR BODY CHEMISTRY

"If someone wishes for good health, one must first ask oneself if he is ready to do away with the reasons for his illness. Only then is it possible to help him."

—Hippocrates

Our bodies truly are designed like magnificent machines. If functioning properly, our cardiovascular system uses a network of arteries, veins, and blood vessels to pump oxygen-rich blood to our vital organs so that they function at maximum capacity. Our lymphatic system also plays a huge role in keeping us healthy by flushing harmful toxins from our body through the liver, lungs, kidneys, intestines, and skin.

However, environmental pollutants, inactivity, and an unhealthy diet can lead to a buildup of toxins in the body. This makes it difficult for our cardiovascular and lymphatic systems to do their jobs properly, which can lead to illnesses such as heart disease, cancer, stroke, diabetes, and infection.

> Our bodies truly are designed like magnificent machines.

Detoxification is vital for cleansing the body of impurities, balancing pH levels, and restoring the circulatory system so that your body can fight off diseases and keep you healthy. Unlike proper nutrition and regular physical activity, which all patients at least have some fundamental knowledge of even if the action or follow-through is not always present, very few are aware that detoxification is a vital and key component of the triad of activities necessary for achieving optimal health and balance.

Over the years, due to cellular breakdown and the accumulation of damaged proteins, as well as the accumulation of ongoing toxins in our technologically driven world, the liver, spleen, blood, and lymphatic systems are overwhelmed and decline in effectiveness and efficiency. This accumulation of toxic material is thought to contribute to cardiovascular and especially neurodegenerative disorders, such as Parkinson's disease.

Some common complaints from my patients include fatigue, headaches, sore backs, digestive problems, and an overall run-down feeling. Lack of energy, aches and pains, and stomach troubles are all signs that there is a buildup of toxins in the body. My recommendation to these clients is a detoxification program.

Despite what many people think, detoxing does not simply involve fasting or drinking strange herbal concoctions. Detoxing is about preventing impurities from entering the body, eliminating the impurities that currently exist, strengthening the lymphatic and cardiovascular systems, and nourishing the body with vital nutrients and minerals. A proper detoxification program aims to restore healthy digestive system function and enhance intrinsic liver detoxification pathways. There are many different ways that you can achieve this.

DETOXIFICATION FOR THE HEART

A RESTORATIVE EFFECT

Maria was forty-two years old. She had Systemic Lupus Erythe-matosus, a long-term autoimmune disease affecting the heart, skin, joints, kidneys, brain, and other organs. She also had three small children and required the help of her sister to care for them.

She was tremendously affected by her disease and needed to spend a portion of the day in bed due to extreme fatigue.

However, after participating in our wellness and detox program, she was able to finally enjoy a full and productive day. Within a matter of weeks, she felt a lifting of her chest pain and body aches, and she had renewed energy. She continues to practice a diet full of green leafy vegetables, a limited intake of refined sugar and processed food, and plenty of alkaline water.

She now understands and is more aware of the importance of taking care of her body and eliminating toxins that exacerbate her condition. Before participating in our wellness program, Maria's body was literally eating itself away and damaging her overall health. Thankfully, she can now enjoy her children with the vigor of a young mother.

Despite eating a healthy diet, toxins can still build up in the body as a result of several external factors like pollution in the air and water, fertilizers and hormones used for growing food, an inactive lifestyle, and even stress. Detoxification is vital for ridding the body of these harmful toxins.

When I suggest detoxification to my patients, many people express concern over the process because they have heard horror stories about fasting, expensive and dubious formulas, and bizarre practices. I tell them to be wary of questionable detox methods. There are many ways to detoxify the body safely and without magic potions or strange procedures.

A good detoxification program involves reducing stress; allowing the organs a chance to rest; cleansing the colon, liver, lungs, kidneys, intestines, and skin of toxins and unnecessary waste products; promoting good circulation; and nourishing the body for more energy and better overall well-being. There are several processes and organ systems that your body uses to detox on a daily basis. The following are some of the best ways to cleanse the body for optimum health.

EXERCISE

Exercise is one of the most important things you can do for your heart, body, and mind. Regular physical activity helps improve overall health and greatly reduces your risk for many chronic diseases. As I discussed in chapter 4, exercise gets the heart rate up, tones the body, lowers blood pressure, reduces stress, and encourages good blood circulation. Also, according to research, exercise is the best thing you can do for your mind to help increase memory and lift depression.

Exercise aids the lymphatic system to remove waste from the body. The lymphatic system is powered by movement, so regular exercise will allow this powerful detoxifying system to eliminate the harmful materials that build up in your body. When you exercise, you are working your lungs, which filter impurities from the air you breathe. A vigorous workout will encourage the sweat to flow, which forces toxins out of the body through the pores. Moreover, exercise reduces fat in the body, which is beneficial for the heart.

Fat binds to toxins within the blood system; therefore the breakdown of fat allows for the toxins to be released, but cleansing and other modalities of elimination are required to remove the toxins from the body. Many types of exercises can assist your body with the detox process. Fitting exercise into your busy schedule may seem difficult, but start slow and engage in physical activities that you enjoy. The following are some great exercises that will help detoxify your body.

Trampoline (Rebounding)

One excellent way to exercise for detoxification is on a mini-trampoline. Also known as rebounding, this type of exercise encourages the lymph to circulate and collect waste in the body. The waste is then expelled from the body through the pores in the skin. The up-and-down motion of rebounding also carries blood to the heart and allows you to breathe deeply so that the lungs can draw in oxygen and expel carbon dioxide and pollutants. Just ten minutes a day of gentle bouncing on a trampoline is enough to encourage detoxification.

George has a history of three vessel bypasses and several stents. Since the birth of his third grandchild, he has taken a new approach to his health. He is realizing at age sixty-eight that he is not invincible and that if he wishes to enjoy a robust life and participate in activities with his grandchildren, he needs to maintain his body in good health.

Luckily, one of George's favorite pastimes is bouncing on the trampoline with his grandchildren. While he might not be able to do the tumbles and the rolls like his four- and six-year-old grandkids do, he is giving his heart, circulation, and lymphatic system a complete overhaul without it seeming like a chore.

This is the best type of exercise that you can incorporate in your daily life: an exercise that you enjoy and that does not feel forced upon you.

This is the best type of exercise that you can incorporate in your daily life: an exercise that you enjoy and does not feel forced upon you.

Yoga

One of the greatest benefits of yoga is its ability to relieve stress. When you are stressed, your body produces hormones that cause the platelets in your blood to stick together. This damages the linings of the artery walls and can lead to strokes and heart attacks. According to an Interheart study, 30 percent of all heart attacks are brought on by stress.

Yoga focuses on deep-breathing techniques, meditation, and gentle stretches and poses that can significantly lower stress levels. In addition, the poses are designed to encourage good circulation and massage the organs. This helps your body to filter out waste materials more efficiently. Hot yoga is particularly good for flushing out toxins, as it causes you to sweat and release toxins through the pores of the skin.

I remember one particular patient, Kimberly, who had originally seen me for chest pain and palpitations. She was working a stressful eighteen-hour-a-day job in the motion picture industry. The stress and demands of her job, the long hours, and the poor eating habits were taking their toll. I urged her to take stock of her life and to reconsider her priorities, and asked if the cost was worth the sacrifice of her mental, emotional, and physical health.

It was a joyous occasion to see her two years later. She looked ten years younger and was vibrant and engaging. She said that she had considered my advice and taken up yoga. It had such a liberating and enlightening effect on her that over one year, she slowly changed her life situation, shifted her career path altogether, and ultimately became a yoga instructor.

Consider the spinal twist, a wonderful detox yoga pose, which assists the lungs with a natural detox process through breathing. This yoga pose has many different variations, but they are all based on the idea that the twisting motion of the spine combined with full deep breaths assists your body in gently clasping and removing toxins from your body.

Now, think of the very popular downward-facing dog position, which is typically used as a resting pose in many yoga sessions. This pose helps with overall circulation and lymph flow and can even aid digestion by incorporating a gentle abdominal stretch.

These yoga poses and many more can be done in a sequence to aid the natural detox process and enhance your body's mental and emotional well-being.

Qigong

Studies show that qigong has a very positive effect on the circulatory system and the removal of waste from the cells of the body. The slow movements in this martial art were designed to allow energy to flow through the body and to remove blockages that can lead to health problems. As I discussed in chapter 4, qigong can also lower blood pressure and promote cardio-vascular health. In addition, this form of exercise reduces stress, which prevents harmful toxins from being released into the bloodstream.

INTERNAL CLEANSING

When most people think of detoxing, they think of cleaning the body from the inside out. Internal cleansing allows the organs to rest and become rejuvenated for better functioning. In addition, a detox diet encourages the body to expel waste materials, a process that flushes toxins out of the system.

There are many ways that you can cleanse your body naturally, including drinking plenty of purified water; eating fresh, organic food that has not been exposed to pesticides or chemicals; consuming herbs that promote liver cleansing, such as green tea and dandelion leaves; cutting out harmful substances such as caffeine and alcohol; and upping your intake of vitamin C to aid the liver in the production of glutathione, which helps force toxins out of the body.

Juice fasting is a popular form of internal cleansing, as it allows your digestive system to rest and clears out waste that has been built up in the intestines.

Although many people report feeling refreshed, energized, and healthier after a detox diet, it is not uncommon to experience some negative side effects from internal cleansing, particularly in the beginning of your detox. Some common side effects include headaches, loss of sleep, skin blemishes, weight loss, irritability, and diarrhea. More often than not, this is your body's reaction to the toxins coming out of your body.

The degree and severity to which your body experiences symptoms is proportionate to the degree of toxins and the level of acidity that exist in your body at the start of the detoxification. These symptoms often clear up after a few days. However, if you experience persistent problems, you may want to consult a doctor or stop the detoxification diet.

HYDROTHERAPY

Water is a powerful detoxifying element for both the inside and outside of our bodies. Hydrotherapy is a method of using water to eliminate toxins in the body. The most popular form of hydrotherapy is the steam bath or sauna. These heated rooms encourage perspiration, which is excellent for opening the pores and pushing toxins out. Steam also helps to clear mucous in the breathing passageways and encourages the lungs to expand and take in more oxygen.

Experts recommend sitting in a steam bath or sauna for no more than fifteen minutes at a time. You will be sweating a lot, so be sure to drink plenty of water to replenish your fluids. In addition, pay attention to your body. If you feel dizzy or faint, leave the heated room and sit down for a few minutes. After your session in the sauna or steam room, be sure to shower to remove the impurities from your skin. It should be noted that saunas and steam baths are not ideal for people who have heart conditions or high blood pressure.

Another form of hydrotherapy is colon hydrotherapy or colonic irrigation. During a typical colonic irrigation session, a therapist will run a small tube through the rectum and into the colon, and then flush water into the colon to soften the stool and eliminate waste and toxins. This has the dual benefit of ridding the digestive tract of harmful bacteria and impurities, and rehydrating the body through the colon. Many people find that they feel lighter, refreshed, and reenergized after a colonic session.

You can also practice hydrotherapy in the comfort of your own home by alternating hot and cold water in the shower. The best way to do this is to stand under hot running water for a few minutes and then switch to a blast of cold water for thirty seconds. Do this three to five times to encourage detoxification.

Hot water opens the pores up and encourages the blood to flow to the surface of the skin, while cold water causes your muscles and pores to restrict, squeezing out impurities and encouraging the blood to flow back toward your vital organs. In this way, you are promoting healthy circulation and eliminating harmful materials from the body.

DRY BRUSHING

Your skin is the largest organ in your body, serving as an important part of the lymphatic system, which removes toxins from the body. Over time, the pores can get clogged with dead skin cells, pollutants, cosmetics, and skin creams. When this happens, your liver and kidneys must work overtime to break down impurities in the body.

Dry brushing is an excellent way to cleanse the pores and remove foreign substances. The best part about dry brushing is that it is inexpensive and easy to do. All you need is a soft brush made with natural fibers. Start by using circular brush strokes on the feet, and slowly move up the legs to the stomach, sides, hands, and arms. Brush in an upward motion toward the heart to encourage good circulation and blood flow.

Dry brushing is especially effective when performed just prior to exercise, a massage, or a sauna bath. After you are done dry brushing the skin, take a shower to remove the impurities from the skin. Many of my patients tell me that their skin feels softer and looks more radiant after dry brushing for just a few days.

I was first introduced to the concept of dry brushing by a massage therapist on a cruise ship. She was from the Philippines and told me that dry brushing is used as a medical therapeutic intervention in her country for people suffering from heart, lung, kidney, and infectious ailments.

MASSAGE

Massages not only feel great, but they can also significantly improve circulation and encourage detoxification. The pressure and kneading sensation of a massage gets the blood flowing, which sends nutrients and oxygen to the organs and helps the organs to expel unnecessary waste. Studies show that massage encourages vasodilation, a condition where the blood vessels expand and blood pressure drops. Moreover, a good massage can relax the body and reduce stress, which is great relief for the cardiovascular and lymphatic systems.

Types of massage include Thai, Balinese, Swedish, hot stone, and hydrotherapy. No matter which style you choose, massages are beneficial for balancing your body chemistry and supporting a healthy heart.

BALANCING YOUR PH: ACIDITY AND ALKALINITY

Very few people are aware that one of the secrets to a healthy heart is your body's pH balance. The cells in your body are constantly emitting acidic waste as a response to energy usage. This acidic waste can seriously damage your cells and vital organs. To neutralize this acidic waste, your body uses nutrients that are alkaline. Ideally, we should be eating a variety of foods that are primarily alkaline so that there is a sufficient store of alkaline material in the body.

Fortunately, the human body is equipped with several mechanisms that work together to maintain pH at an optimal level. Our healthy organs are able to neutralize and eliminate excess acid from the body—but within limits. If you have low levels of alkaline nutrients from food, the body will take nutrients from other important areas, such as the bones. Also, since fat is a great buffer for acidity, having an imbalance of more acidic food intake will lead to more fat storage.

The pH scale ranges from 0 to 14, with 0 to 7 being acidic and 7 to 14 being alkaline. A healthy pH level for the blood is 7.4. Acidosis is a condition where the blood is too acidic, and this can expose the body to increased risk of several health problems such as heart disease, arthritis, cancer, and diabetes.

When the blood is too acidic, the body's cells begin to die and cannot regenerate. This means that your body cannot take in the nutrients it needs or eliminate toxins. A buildup of acidity prevents your organs from functioning properly, thickens the blood, and starts to dissolve the linings of the arteries. This causes strain on the heart and can lead to cardiovascular disease.

In addition, most cancer cells thrive in an acidic environment. Inflammatory disease, arthritis, respiratory conditions, and cardiovascular diseases are also more prevalent in an acidic environment. High acidic levels in the body lead to severe damage of the inner lining of the blood vessels. In fact, cholesterol can be thought of as bandages that provide healing to the acid-burned areas of the blood vessel. However, continued damage to the inner lining of the blood vessel leads to the formation of atherosclerotic plaque within the arteries.

Maintaining a healthy pH balance is very important. The best way to maintain an adequate acid-alkaline body balance is by consuming a healthy diet composed of at least 80 percent alkaline foods and limiting highly acidic foods.

Acidic foods include red and white meats, dairy, refined sugars and artificial sweeteners, processed foods, white flour, oysters, shrimp, coffee, soft drinks, and alcohol. The standard Western diet today is primarily composed of highly acidic foods, which overwhelm the body's natural mechanisms for removing excess acid, making us more susceptible to illness and disease. Our diets are very notably deficient in alkalinizing natural foods.

Eat more alkaline whole foods and discover a wide range of health benefits and longevity. A healthy, well-balanced diet should consist mostly of alkaline foods, such as:

- Vegetables: green salads, avocados, artichokes, asparagus, broccoli, cabbage, carrots, celery, cucumbers, garlic, kale, leeks, mushrooms, onions, peas, peppers, spinach, squash, tomatoes, zucchini

- Fruits: apples, bananas, cantaloupes, grapes, grapefruits, lemons and limes, peaches

- Seeds, nuts, and grains: pumpkin, sesame, flax, sunflower, buckwheat, almonds

- Natural fats and oils: olive, flax

- Drinks: water, herbal teas, fresh vegetable juices, non-sweetened soy milk

WATER

Jan was a patient of mine who came to me with complaints of daily fatigue, nausea, and dizziness. We ran tests to see if we could identify the problem, but nothing out of the ordinary showed up. Jan was baffled because she lived a healthy lifestyle. She did not smoke or drink excessively. She exercised regularly and ate her fair share of fruits, vegetables, protein, and grains. At one point I asked her to keep a food diary to see if we could pinpoint the cause of her symptoms.

When Jan brought her diary in for me to analyze, I immediately noticed the problem. Although Jan's diet consisted of healthy foods, she rarely drank water. Other than a small glass of juice or coffee with her meals, Jan was essentially running on empty when it came to her fluid intake and hydration.

I urged Jan to drink a large glass of water with every meal and at least one glass of water between every meal. Lo and behold, within a few days the symptoms had cleared up and Jan felt a better sense of well-being. The moral of the story is to never underestimate the power of a simple glass of water.

In contrast, Mark is a water maven. He has hypertension, palpitations, and minor blockages of his blood vessels. On his recent visit, he told me that he had made a substantial investment in a water ionization system. He had done it for his twelve-year-old son, who had been diagnosed with lymphoma. While the initial investment was solely for the sake of warding off the cancer from raging in his young son's body, he has noticed appreciable changes in himself.

The most notable positive change was that he had never before been a water drinker, but once he started drinking the alkaline water, he became more and more drawn to drinking water. He limited other beverages, as if his body woke up and recognized the vital life-enhancing molecule that he had been lacking. He noticed a greater calmness and feeling of well-being, and surprisingly his blood pressure began to decrease. Better yet, he managed to effortlessly shed ten pounds just by drinking alkaline water.

Water is the top life-giving element for all living beings. Scientists estimate that a healthy person could go a number of weeks without food, provided that he or she had plenty of water. However, after just a few days without water, that same person would perish from dehydration. Water supports every system in our body, and it is essential for good health.

Clean, pure water is vital for several reasons. It helps flush out toxins through the liver and the kidneys; transports nutrients throughout the bloodstream; regulates pH levels, metabolism, and body temperature; and lubricates the joints. Without water, our bodies become

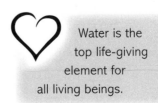
Water is the top life-giving element for all living beings.

dehydrated, which can cause the heart to beat irregularly and the blood vessels to constrict, preventing proper blood circulation. Dehydration is a very dangerous condition that could lead to death.

The human body is composed of 60 to 80 percent water, with the highest percentage of body weight seen in a newborn and then steadily declining with age. So it is no wonder that we can easily become dehydrated if we do not successfully replenish our daily loss of water, which occurs through our breath, perspiration, and urine and bowel elimination. It is estimated that 75 percent of Americans are chronically dehydrated.

This takes a tremendous toll on our health and on our vital organs, when one considers that 85 percent of the brain, 80 percent of the blood, and 70 percent of our lean muscle are composed of water.

The Institute of Medicine suggests that people in good health should drink nine cups of water daily to stay hydrated. In general, the appropriate recommendation is to drink your lean body weight in ounces, or 0.6 to 0.7 ounces per pound of total body weight. Of course, the amount of water you need to drink depends on a number of factors, including the condition of your health, activity level, and the climate you live in.

On any given day we lose about 2.5 liters of water just by going about our regular routine. This number increases when you add exercise and heat into the mix. A good way to make sure you are getting enough water is to drink enough so that you are not thirsty and your urine is clear or pale yellow. People with heart conditions should be careful about the amount of water they drink, as excess drinking of water could cause fluid retention, which can stress the cardiovascular system.

Another thing to consider is the pH level of the water you drink. Alkaline, or ionized water, is better for our bodies because it can reduce harmful acidity in the body and eliminate toxins. Certain foods that we eat can cause our bodies to become too acidic, which can lead to many health problems. Ionized water can help to rebalance the pH levels in the body.

Water that is between 8.5 and 9.0 pH is considered alkaline. You can check the pH level of your water with a pH testing strip. If your water is too acidic, you may want to consider an alkaline water ionizer, alkaline tablets, or alkaline drops. I myself have an alkalinizing machine, and I feel that it has added value to the health of my family.

AVOID FOODS THAT WREAK HAVOC ON YOUR HEART

We all know that certain foods are good for us and others are bad, but many people do not understand exactly which foods are bad for our health and why. Foods containing trans fats, saturated fats, cholesterol, salt, and sugars can all negatively affect the way the body functions.

Over time, a buildup of these harmful substances can deposit toxins in the bloodstream, cells, and intestinal tract, and can contribute to clogged arteries, heart attacks, diabetes, and strokes. It is important to be aware of the foods that contain these substances so you can make healthy eating choices.

Saturated Fats and Trans Fats

Numerous studies have proven that the consumption of saturated fats is directly linked to heart disease, hypertension, and strokes. Saturated fats are found mainly in animal products, and they are made up of triglycerides that are completely saturated with fatty acids.

When you consume foods that contain saturated fats, your body produces more bad LDL cholesterol, which begins to build up in your arteries. This prevents the blood from flowing properly to the heart, and can result in heart attacks and strokes.

Trans fats are even worse for your body, as they raise LDL cholesterol and lower good HDL cholesterol. Saturated fats and trans fats can be found in animal products such as meat, butter, cheese, and milk, as well as coconut oil, palm oil, pastries, cookies, and cakes. The AHA suggests limiting your intake of saturated and trans fats to less than 7 percent of your total diet.

Sodium

Salt may make meals taste better, but too much salt in the diet can be dangerous. Our bodies need a minimal amount of sodium to manage fluid levels, conduct electricity in the nervous system, and encourage proper muscle function. However, studies show that excessive salt consumption is directly related to hypertension.

Too much salt in the body causes water retention and increases blood volume. This means that your heart has to work harder to pump blood throughout the body. People who consume too much salt run the risk of developing heart disease and kidney disease.

Perhaps the best example of the benefits of lowering salt intake comes from Finland. Thirty years ago, the government of Finland started strongly promoting diets that were low in salt. Over the decades, the Finnish people collectively lowered their salt intake by 33 percent. As a result, deaths from coronary heart disease and stroke have declined by 75 to 80 percent.

The AHA recommends limiting salt intake to less than 1,500 milligrams a day. You can lower your salt intake by avoiding processed foods, checking the labels on the foods you buy, and replacing salt as a food enhancer with healthy herbs and spices. You will also want to be mindful when eating certain ethnic foods, such as Japanese sushi, Chinese food, Korean food, and Indian food, as well as canned or frozen foods.

Sugar

It is a well-known fact that eating large quantities of sugar can lead to weight gain. What many people do not realize is that foods that are high in sugar can also cause diabetes and cardiovascular disease. Sugar causes an increase in blood glucose levels, bad LDL cholesterol, and trigylcerides. A study called the Coronary Artery Risk in Young Adults showed that high-sugar diets can negatively affect the levels of good HDL cholesterol in the blood.

One of the best things you can do for your heart is to reduce the amount of refined sugars in your diet. Refined sugar goes by many names, including sucrose, fructose, dextrose, and glucose. By reading the labels of packaged food, you can avoid consuming more sugars than necessary.

The USDA recommends limiting sugar to less than eight teaspoons a day. Also be aware that four grams of carbohydrates are equivalent to one teaspoon of sugar. Therefore, a typical glass of orange juice, which contains approximately twenty-eight grams of carbohydrates, is adding seven teaspoons of sugar to your daily intake. People with heart disease and diabetes should not only avoid refined sugars, but should also be mindful of their intake of healthy fruit.

Cholesterol

We need cholesterol in our bodies to produce hormones, create new cells, and support the nervous system. However, there are two types of cholesterol: LDL cholesterol, which is bad for your health; and HDL cholesterol, which is the good kind.

When oxidized LDL cholesterol builds up in the arteries, it results in a condition called atherosclerosis. Arteries that are clogged with this waxy substance prevent the heart from transporting nutrient-rich blood to the vital organs. This strains the heart and can lead to congestive heart failure and cardiovascular disease. HDL cholesterol, on the other hand, helps to clear the bad cholesterol from the body.

Our liver produces about 75 percent of the cholesterol in our bodies, and we get the remaining 25 percent from the food we eat. Cholesterol is found in animal products such as meat, butter, cheese, and milk. The best way to cut back on the amount of cholesterol you eat is by avoiding red meat and dairy products.

Caffeine and Alcohol

If you are like most of my patients, you start the day with a cup of coffee or tea to jumpstart your brain. However, research shows that caffeine can increase your risk of heart disease. A study at the Duke University Medical Center showed that people who consumed caffeine experienced a dramatic spike in blood pressure that lasted for a number of hours. In addition, those same people had a 32 percent increase in stress hormone levels after consuming caffeine. Experts agree that cutting back on caffeine can help to ward off hypertension and cardiovascular disease.

In terms of alcohol, studies show that a moderate amount of alcohol (one to two drinks per day) can benefit the heart and reduce your risk of developing heart disease and diabetes. The National Institute on Alcohol Abuse and Alcoholism (NIAAA) even reports that moderate drinkers have the greatest longevity.

Possible reasons for these benefits may include improvement in the blood lipid profile, a decrease in blood clotting, a decrease in coronary vasospasm, an increase in coronary blood flow, a reduction in blood pressure, a reduction in insulin levels, and an increase in estrogen levels.

Despite these beneficial effects, as a general rule I don't recommend alcohol to my patients as a form of treatment. As a whole, alcohol has too much potential for turning into an abusive habit, and excessive alcohol intake can have a detrimental effect on the body and on the mind.

When you drink alcohol, it is filtered through your liver and passed through your kidneys. Excess alcohol consumption causes these detoxifying organs to work overtime, which in turn prevents the body from filtering other toxins efficiently. The standard rule is that one glass of alcohol a day is fine, but anything more than that can lead to serious health problems.

The methods of detoxification that you choose are entirely up to you. I recommend detoxifying the body once or twice a year in order to clear out any buildup of toxins and to realign your body chemistry.

Before undergoing any type of detox, it is important to consult with your physician or health-care professional. Detox is not for everyone, and it can be dangerous for some individuals—especially pregnant women, nursing mothers, small children, the elderly, and those with chronic health conditions. A doctor can give you sound advice about whether detox is right for you, and if so, which methods are best suited to your lifestyle and health condition.

MIND-BODY AXIS

MENTAL, EMOTIONAL, AND SPIRITUAL DETOXIFICATION

There are three aspects of mental, emotional, and spiritual (MES) detoxification that are critical to obtaining optimal health.

First, it is important to be able to minimize or eliminate stress, anxiety, and fear in our daily routine. We live in a stressful, fearful world. People feel the need to protect themselves and often let fear eclipse common sense. Fear is an irrational part of a negative belief system, an expectation that the worst will happen.

How do we effectively minimize stress, anxiety, and fear? Quite simply, we change our outlook or perception on circumstances. There are always going to be circumstances in our lives that pose challenges; the manner in which we perceive these challenges as either stepping stones to elevate our growth or obstacles that are intentionally placed in our path to defeat us can have a tremendous impact on the neurotransmitters and signals released in our bodies. These neuro-pathways will either boost or weaken our immune system, our cardiovascular system, and our entire body.

One simple exercise is to practice being grateful. Gratitude enhances your sense of happiness and well-being. Gratitude and appreciation for all that you have, both the good and the bad, have the power to transform the way you live your life and the manner in which you manifest your health. So start each morning with a list of five things you are grateful for that day.

The second important MES detoxification process is to eliminate the feeling of lack. Too many of us have this notion

that outside circumstances control our happiness, relationships, time, money, freedom, and health. "If only my job were not so stressful, if only I had more time, if only my aching knees would allow me to exercise, if only they would serve healthy food at work, if only…"

As long as we hold the belief that we have "lack" in our lives due to circumstances outside of our control, we will never be truly "rich" in health, or in any other aspect of our lives. One detox practice that minimizes the feeling of lack or constriction is to be giving, freely, of your time and money.

The final MES detox is to practice forgiveness. Forgiveness is by far the most potent MES detoxification that you can practice. Forgiveness allows for a shift in our perception, which is necessary for our emotional, mental, and spiritual growth and healing. Forgiveness liberates us from constriction and frees us to live in balance. Forgiveness is for ourselves. Forgiveness evokes healing, as in the case of Lester Levenson, who I write about in chapter 10.

Healing is truly about relationships—with self and with all of those around us. Health comes out of improved relationships—love of self and self-esteem, intimacy with others, and unity with a higher being. One cannot be truly healthy unless one has practiced forgiveness and released the negative emotional vibratory signals that come out of self-deprecation or hatred and anger toward others.

A simple act of forgiveness is to bless all who cross our path and to see only goodness in them and wish them well. In doing these simple acts of kindness, we are liberating ourselves to embody radiant health.

CHAPTER 6

REVIVE YOUR EMOTIONAL HEART

"Why do two colors, put one next to the other, sing? Can one really explain this?"

—Pablo Picasso

What does the term "renewable energy" mean to you? We hear a lot about escalating demands for energy, high levels of consumption, and environmental concerns around the use of nonrenewable fossil fuels. There is a strong movement toward finding alternative energy sources, such as solar, wind, and wave power.

Have you ever thought of renewable energy in the context of what fuels our bodies? We need incredible amounts of energy to sustain our daily lives. Where does that energy come from? What fuels our mind, body, and spirit? What is the energy source that keeps our heart beating?

We can learn about one source of renewable energy by watching the way children respond to life. No matter how much energy children expend, they always have more.

Children love to run for no particular reason and to no particular destination.

> Children are fed by a powerful energy source called "joie de vivre," the French expression for joy of living.

They run for the joy of feeling the breeze, for the excitement of feeling their small hearts pumping, and for the feel of the solid earth pounding beneath their feet. Children love to explore and climb. They clamber up trees, swing from branches, and hang upside down. They never tire of playing.

As parents and caregivers, we often wonder where all that energy comes from. It's not simply that children are young, without the aches and pains of aging. Children are fed by a powerful energy source called "joie de vivre," the French expression for joy of living. Children have an unbridled joie de vivre. They don't think about the hows or whys. They are energized by life itself.

As we grow older, the stresses of life can sap our joie de vivre. We lose our ability to sustain ourselves with the joy of life. Instead we turn to quick energy that gets us through the day but does not sustain us over the long term. We function with stress, and at times we even seem to thrive on stress.

Stress is part of a biological state of arousal of our sympathetic nervous system called the fight-or-flight response. In evolutionary terms, stress plays an essential role in our survival. It is intended to keep us safe from harm by preparing us to either flee from danger or gather resources to fight.

When presented with a threat, a number of physiological responses occur: heartbeat and breathing speed up, blood vessels constrict, and various nonessential processes slow or halt. Your body prepares for action by diverting all physiological resources into fight-or-flight mode and suppressing unnecessary activities.

We are flooded with adrenaline, which causes the heart to beat faster, constricts the muscles, and causes us to breathe deeply. Adrenaline gives us surges of energy and heightens our sensory awareness. The body also produces cortisol, a hormone that increases glucose in the bloodstream and temporarily stops the digestive and immune systems from functioning.

Not only does the stress response prepare us to meet challenges, it can also provide an energy source. Stress can give us the motivation to succeed, similar to an athlete who wants to finish first in the race. Stress hormones provide positive outcomes in the short term, but they do not last and must be constantly replaced.

> Stress is part of a biological state of arousal of our sympathetic nervous system called the fight-or-flight response.

A healthy diet and regular exercise are the basic physical sources of energy, easily renewed and essential to sustaining life. Unfortunately, we have become accustomed to using stress and adrenaline as a fuel source, and we often replace the quality energy sources of exercise and diet with cheap alternative sources such as junk food, caffeine, nicotine, and activities that give us an adrenaline high.

When prolonged bouts of stress—or the need to maintain a condition of readiness to fight or flee—set in, the physical body suffers. A negative consequence of the fight-or-flight response is the suppression of the physiological processes our body considers unnecessary during fleeing or fighting, including the digestive system, sexual responses, and the immune system.

Over an extended period, this immune suppression will lead to a host of stress-related illnesses, including heart disease, diabetes, chronic fatigue, anxiety, depression, insomnia, sexual problems, stomach ailments, and much more. Studies show that people who have high levels of cortisol and adrenaline are at a much higher risk of developing hypertension, atherosclerosis, cardiomyopathy, coronary heart disease, diabetes, and cancer.

According to the AHA, chronic stress raises the heart rate and blood pressure, which can damage the walls of your arteries. In addition, people who are chronically stressed may overeat or handle difficult situations by smoking or drinking heavily, which can lead to dangerous health conditions. Longitudinal studies have revealed that ongoing stress can even

To become and remain healthy, we must build sustainable and renewable energy sources that will revitalize our heart, mind, and soul.

destroy brain cells, hinder learning and memory, and perhaps alter our very DNA. It is no wonder that stress-related illness forms the bulk of most doctor referrals. It is certainly a contributing factor in many of my cardiac evaluations.

Using the stress response as fuel provides energy in the short term, but it is not healthy or sustainable over a long period. Our nutritional reserves and blood sugar levels become depleted and we burn out quickly. Chronic stress conditions can seriously harm our health, taking an incredible toll on our bodies and our immune systems.

Yet many have become addicted to the short rush of adrenaline energy, rather than to building sustainable energy reserves. We live increasingly stressful lives, often not noticing the toll it takes on our health until it is too late. Until a few years ago, that described my life. I thrived on challenges, and multitasking was my mantra. As I shared earlier, that resulted in a breakdown in my personal life.

Research studies performed at Stanford and other centers have shown that multitasking leads to increased stress, lack of focus, memory lapse, decreased productivity, impaired learning, and blunted creativity.

To become and remain healthy, we must build sustainable and renewable energy sources that will revitalize our heart, mind, and soul. We need to make lifestyle changes and adjust our attitude toward strengthening and nourishing our heart. We need to learn to stay focused and on task, practice mindfulness, and be present in the moment. How, then, do we achieve these goals and find renewable and sustainable energy sources for the long term?

Let's consider some of the renewable energy sources that will revive your emotional heart: love, laughter, creativity, and music.

THOU SHALT LOVE: WHO?

DANCING ATTENDANCE ON HEALTH

Linda loved to dance. She lived for weekly dance classes, when she could put on her jazz slippers, stretch her muscles, and move across the room to the music, feeling graceful and beautiful. She would disappear into the dance and let the movement and the music take her away from everything else in the world.

Although surrounded by mirrors in the studio, Linda didn't seem to notice that she was extremely overweight. Instead, she saw the artistic line of her arm, the elastic power of her muscles, the strength of each pirouette, the wonderful rhythm that coursed through her body.

At the age of fifteen, Linda performed a lyrical dance on stage. She wore a beautiful, white lycra dress with a tight bodice and flowing skirt that she loved. It whirled around her body as she spun across the stage, expressing every passionate note in the lines of her body. She loved the choreography and she poured all her emotion into each movement, losing herself in the dance as it nurtured her soul.

Back in the dressing room, Linda stood smiling in front of the mirror in her flowing lycra dress, still feeling the warm glow of her performance. Suddenly she heard laughter and low voices from a group of girls in the next room. "She looked like a beached whale flopping in distress!" they giggled. "Didn't her mother see how ridiculous she looked in that white dress? She was like a giant sailboat!"

Linda looked in the mirror and suddenly saw her body for what it really was: fat, ugly, disgusting. Consumed with self-hatred, Linda tore off the dress and left in tears.

For years Linda punished herself by eating. She hated her body. She was ugly and she just wanted to eat her way into oblivion. At university, Linda found herself drawn to the counseling field, working with children who had experienced early trauma. In exploring possible therapies, Linda remembered how good dancing had made her feel, how the music had energized her. One day she pulled out her old ballet slippers and went to a drop-in class. Her body still looked large and heavy in the mirror, but as soon as Linda donned the shoes, she felt light and thin as air.

At that moment, Linda knew what she had to do. To bring dance back into her life, she needed to start loving her body. Linda had another powerful motivation. She had grown up with two obese parents who smoked and drank heavily. A family history of heart disease and hypertension had contributed to the early deaths of several close relatives. When Linda looked in the mirror, she realized that years of self-hatred toward her body were leading her down a dangerous path.

Linda visited me, and together we planned a diet, exercise, and wellness regimen that would help her lose weight quickly and safely. Dance was to be the central point and motivator. Daily dance classes and artistic workouts were supplemented by yoga and meditation to help her remain focused.

Within a year, Linda had met her target weight and had become a stellar model of healthy living. Her risk of heart disease had normalized.

Linda invited me to her year-end dance performance. She again performed a flowing, lyrical piece. As she gracefully moved across the stage, feeling empowered and energized with a new sense of health and well-being, I realized that something important had changed for Linda. Dance was no longer simply a refuge or an escape. Linda's love of dance had shown her a way to love herself. Linda was now actively expressing that love, through dance.

L-O-V-E: a simple word that evokes a powerful emotional, mental, and physical response. We sing about love. We write books and poetry dedicated to love. We create beautiful works of art and sculpture to express love. Love is the main topic in virtually all creative art forms and has been expressed artistically in every culture and language since the dawn of time. It can be defined as a strong emotional attachment toward another person or thing. Love is linked with intimacy, but it is also a vital social bond that connects us with others.

However, showing love toward others is not enough. All too often, we focus our love on others, neglecting ourselves in the process. If we want to achieve heart health and emotional wellness, love of self must be part of the process.

It is human nature to take good care of the things we love, whether they are people or possessions. If you love yourself, you will take care of yourself. You are less likely to engage in self-harming and unhealthy behaviors, such as overeating, alcohol abuse, or harmful excess of any kind. You will make sure you get sufficient rest, and you will allow your body to recuperate from stress. If you love yourself, you will take time to nurture your soul with creative pursuits and activities that bring you happiness and satisfaction.

Loving yourself will make you more lovable and more able to love others. It is

> L-O-V-E: a simple word that evokes a powerful emotional, mental, and physical response.

> If we want to achieve heart health and emotional wellness, love of self must be part of the process.

especially important that you learn to love your body, as that vibration syncs up with creating a body that you love, because you will not stay in a body that you do not love.

To love and be loved is a core human need. Interpersonal love in a relationship is important, but filling our lives with love involves much more. It includes love we show for others, whether it be a partner, our children, friends, the community, or God. It includes charitable love expressed through hospitality or good deeds. It includes love of beauty, art, and virtue. Most importantly, it involves love of self.

If we feel every type of love toward ourselves, emotionally and physically, and if we build on each type of love and show it toward others, we will revitalize our heart and become healthy—with love.

MUSIC, DANCE, AND CREATIVITY

Music, dance, and creativity are all effective ways to access inner energy sources and revitalize our hearts. The power music exerts is undeniable, yet the appeal cannot be explained in evolutionary terms. Music, dance, and other creative pursuits have no apparent survival value. They do not satisfy hunger, make us more attractive sexually, or help us live longer.

Yet creativity, art, music, and dance are an essential part of every culture and have been since the beginning of history. We are drawn to music and dance, both as spectators and as participants. We surround ourselves with artistic beauty and creativity.

Music and dance are creative pursuits that are particularly good for our heart health because they have both emotional and physical benefits. They allow easy participation, even for those who may feel they lack artistic talent. We can use music and dance to get in touch with our inner self, to learn to love our physical body. While it may seem to have no survival function, in reality music plays a key role in our survival by positively impacting our health and wellness.

Dance Me to the End of Love

When disco music first took the world by storm in the 1970s, many theories were advanced as to its popularity. One of the most convincing was the premise that disco music mimicked the heartbeat exactly. This theory became so widely accepted that disco music became the preferred CPR aid for helping emergency responders create and remember the proper rhythm for compressions within the range of 100 to 120 beats a minute.

"Stayin' Alive" by the Bee Gees, at 102 beats per minute, has been the song of choice for CPR training for many years. The sentiment of the tune no doubt helps with the task. The idea that rhythm and music appeals to the beat of our heart is an important one.

Drum rhythms have a proven power that has been used for centuries in traditional medicine. Rhythm moves us physically, motivating a desire to dance. Increasingly, researchers are recognizing the importance of dance to physical and emotional health. Not only is dance a fun and effective way to exercise, it increases brain chemicals that encourage nerve cell growth, improves memory skills, and triggers a mind-body connection.

Dancing is effective therapy for dementia and Alzheimer's disease, osteoporosis, and diabetes. It helps restore physical mobility for individuals with brain injury or Parkinson's patients, and it enhances physical therapy. Dancing improves heart health, reduces blood pressure, and lowers stress. Dancing is an effective tool to combat obesity and improve physical fitness, especially in the sedentary adolescent population.

THE RHYTHM OF LONGEVITY

Consider the case study of Margaret, an eighty-nine-year-old woman who loved to line dance. She had been dancing every Wednesday at her senior community center for years. Line dancing sustained her and energized her without the physical demands of a workout. It also provided a sense of friendship and community.

Margaret had critical aortic stenosis, which is the narrowing of the main valve out of the chamber of the heart. Normally the opening is about the size of a silver dollar (3 cm), but Margaret's had narrowed to less than the size of a dime (0.8 cm). The diminished blood flow caused difficult symptoms and led to her being hospitalized with congestive heart failure (fluid in the lungs due to backflow of blood from the heart).

An aortic valve replacement surgery was recommended, but Margaret resisted, insisting that she wanted to leave this earth as she arrived—with all her organs intact.

Indignant at her refusal, the surgeon, backed by her cardiologist, gave Margaret only six months to live. Margaret did not care for this scare tactic and discharged herself from the hospital. She came to me for a second opinion.

I advised her that statistically the diagnosis was correct, since the survival rate for people with critical aortic stenosis declines sharply once congestive heart failure develops. However, I did validate her assumption that statistics were simply an approximation and that with all statistical data there was always individual variability. Margaret, having been prepared for only six months more of life without the surgery, was pleased to hear that she might have longer than that.

With her strong will and desire to live, and armed with the belief that her physical condition would not limit her, Margaret kept dancing every Wednesday. Six months came and went, and Margaret did not stop dancing.

I managed Margaret's care for the next five years, during which she continued to defy science and challenge the statistics. Although she had some physical limitations and symptoms of shortness of breath, she had no further hospitalization from congestive heart failure or chest symptoms. Even with small physical declines, she remained vibrant in mind and spirit.

After five years I handed Margaret's care to another cardiologist when I left my practice in Santa Monica. It is my hope that Margaret is still dancing every Wednesday at the senior community center.

Margaret combined a positive attitude toward life with her love of an artistic pursuit. This enabled her to not only survive far longer than statistically predicted, but also to enjoy her life in a way that defied science. Her love of dance helped motivate her, and the physical benefits of dance helped keep her healthy. For anyone, at any age, learning to dance can fill a necessary emotional need and heal the heart.

My Heart's Rhythm

A popular yearly music festival takes place on traditional native lands in a remote valley in northern Canada. Families set up tents for the weekend and enjoy a celebration of music and life — rain or shine. The festival is held in mid-June, and the weather can be markedly chilly, but the music and the camaraderie keep things warm.

Along the pathway to the four stages where the professional musicians perform, a series of tarps marks one very special area—the community drum circle. Throughout the weekend, a group is always playing drums under the tarps, nonstop, day and night. People of all ages pass by and pause, pick up one of the many drums available, and join in.

There is an incredible sense of peace and companionship, a linking of heartbeats and spirits for a moment. Each beat resonates and echoes into the valley. Some keep a regular rhythm, while others take turns expressing a particular emotion or sharing a personal rhythmic anthem. The drum circle both energizes the festival and imbues a sense of calm. It is a place of peace and rejuvenation.

When we hear a rhythm, almost invariably we find ourselves moving with the beat, tapping toes or fingers. A phenomenon called brainwave entrainment occurs, whereby our heartbeat and brain waves begin to match the rhythm. Researchers are beginning to study this incredibly powerful response, seeing potential in it for a range of medical treatments.

There are indications that these rhythms stimulate brain neurotransmitters such as endorphins and dopamine, which are related to emotional regulation. Initial studies have shown promise for treatment of anxiety, depression, Parkinson's disease, pain control, and a number of other ailments.

Drums and rhythm are simple and basic ways to energize our hearts. Drum circles are defined as a way for a group of people to gather in a circle to express themselves with drums and percussion. Although drum circles have been used traditionally for centuries, in recent years therapists and clinicians have started to incorporate drum circles into many health applications.

Corporations use drum circles for team building, employee wellness, personal empowerment, and workplace stress. Therapists and healthcare professionals use drum circles in addiction treatment, trauma treatment, and other clinical interventions, in working with persons with disabilities, and for stress reduction and wellness. Drumming and rhythm are incredibly powerful therapeutic tools that can serve as a renewable energy source.

How can you use a drum circle for heart health? You don't need "real" drums. Any kind of surface will do. Start with a heartbeat—one, two, three, four. Each person in the circle first joins the communal beat, then takes a turn at expressing his or her own rhythm. As you follow the beat and let yourself go into the rhythm of the heart, you will find it easy to let daily cares drift away.

Social bonds and community inclusion are fostered through drum circles, but individually within the circle we also experience personal empowerment, stress reduction, a strengthened immune system, emotional release, and better heart health.

Drumming and rhythm can also be used individually as an aid to meditation. Keeping a rhythmic pattern creates a mantra that will help you relax and focus. The deliberation and sound of the drum beat help you clear your mind of worries and negative thoughts.

As you attend to the rhythm, you become aware of your breathing and connect with your heartbeat. Your brain waves slow, and your body relaxes. Drumming meditation can bring you into a heightened state of awareness and help you get in touch with your own creative rhythms inside. Drumming connects you to your heartbeat. Drumming keeps you present in the moment.

MUSIC HEALS THE HEART

I have known Joe for years, helping him manage his blood pressure and life stressors. His blood pressure and other symptoms always fluctuated with his mood, and the slightest ailment would distress him. Joe experienced intermittent chest pain, making necessary numerous evaluations. Fortunately, none of the tests revealed any cardiac pathology.

On a recent visit, Joe seemed different, more serene. I had not seen him in over a year, and when I inquired, he informed me that he had been battling prostate cancer and had undergone chemotherapy and surgery. Knowing how stress had always affected him, I asked how he was handling this health issue. Surprisingly, Joe stated that he was doing very well, which was verified by his blood pressure and pulse.

Joe explained that because of his illness, he had retired from his business and was now devoting his spare time to his greatest and first love—music. Joe is a proficient jazz musician and had gotten together with his old band members, who were all retirement-aged. Joe and his band perform weekly at a local nightclub.

As Joe spoke about music and reminisced about jazz halls and music clubs, the energy of the room lifted and changed from sorrow over his cancer diagnosis to a mood of love, joy, and entertainment. It was clear that rediscovering his love for music had sustained Joe in his fight against cancer, and his blood pressure and chest symptoms had not been an issue since he had begun to regularly play jazz music again.

Given Joe's history of dealing with stress, his cancer diagnosis might well have taken him down a very different path. Instead, his attitude toward a negative event was one of gratitude . . . gratitude for his life, for his music, for his physicians, and for his treatment. This feeling of gratitude shifted his vibrational energy and allowed him to reconnect with his divine spirit and rediscover his inner love of music. He now uses creativity and music to heal his heart and reshape his life, taking it in a new direction.

How can music be a source of energy and healing in our lives? We may not be professional jazz musicians like Joe, but we can use music and dance to our benefit in countless ways. Simply listening to music can have a relaxing, calming effect when we feel stressed. If we are tired and finding it difficult to be motivated to action, music can energize us.

The best way to benefit from music and dance, however, is to actively participate. Drums are an easy way to start, but there are many other ways to become involved in music, rhythm, and dance. If you've played an instrument or been involved in dance at a previous time in your life, explore the possibility of renewing that relationship.

Formal classes in music or dance are always a possibility, but many communities also host informal dance groups. You can enjoy the empowering benefits of music and dance even if you are dancing alone in your room. There are many options and possibilities. Choose one and make music and dance part of your life.

Traveling to the Beat of a Different Drum

"If a man loses pace with his companions, perhaps it is because he hears a different drummer."

—Henry David Thoreau

Traveling to the beat of a different drum and the expression "march to a different drummer" are both familiar terms. Most people understand them to mean you are embracing a personal philosophy or idea that may differ from someone else's.

Beating a different drum takes courage and it often causes people to fear isolation. Yet why should you fear being different from the crowd? Is acceptance really that important? Is it healthier to follow the crowd, or do we achieve greater energy by following our own unique heart's desire?

Becoming comfortable with following your own drum goes back to learning how to love yourself. If you can celebrate the person inside you that travels to that different rhythm, you will have the confidence you need to follow the drumbeat.

MAKING A MUSICAL CHOICE

Aaron was a talented musician and singer with an unusual, powerful voice that spanned several octaves. At the encouragement of friends, he entered a major talent contest. Although he did not win, agents and record companies noticed. Soon Aaron was presented with several lucrative recording deals and the opportunity to be the opening act for a major rock-and-roll artist.

Aaron had been raised by his mother as part of a devout religious group that considered rock music harmful. She did not want him to follow a career in music, but instead desired for him to devote himself to his faith. Trying to please his mother, Aaron turned down all the recording opportunities. As the weeks and months passed, he found himself becoming increasingly despondent. It became difficult to get out of bed in the morning, and soon he could not even find solace in music.

His younger sister encouraged Aaron to follow his heart and, without his knowledge, posted a video of him singing on YouTube. Agents again noticed Aaron's talent and started calling. Aaron's mother delivered an ultimatum. If he chose the professional music world, she would disown him. Aaron was deeply torn, but his sister encouraged him not to give up on his dream. Remembering how horrible he had felt without his music, Aaron decided he could not continue to live his mother's dream but had to follow his own.

As Aaron sang on stage, sharing his talent and his love of music with thousands of fans, his heart filled with a joy and profound fulfillment he'd never thought possible. It had been painful, but he knew he had made the right decision.

Most of us will never face such an extreme choice, but we all have pressures that interfere with our freedom to choose the direction we want our life to take. Those pressures may be tangible, such as a lack of money, family responsibilities, or physical limitations; or they may be internal factors such as fear of displeasing a parent, lack of self-confidence, or intimidation by pressure from peers, a social group, or our religious upbringing.

Oftentimes we face choices between competing desires, both of which may appeal to some aspect of ourselves. How, then, do we follow our own drummer when we aren't quite sure which is the best way to go?

One way to make the right choices regarding the direction of our lives is to think about life in the context of death. You are no doubt pursuing the secrets to your vibrant heart because you want to live a long, healthy life. You want to live that life to the fullest, feeling energized in mind, body, soul, and spirit. So ask yourself: "If today were the last day of my life, would I want to be doing what I have planned?" Would you choose to live that day meeting the expectations of other people? Or would you have the courage to follow your heart?

Traveling to the beat of your own drum is an important part of learning ways to energize your heart. Don't let the thinking and opinions of other people obscure your inner voice. You are working hard to become energized and healthy, so align your goals and perspectives with the person you want to become. Don't waste another day living someone else's life. Live your own.

LAUGHTER AND HEART HEALTH

WHEN LUCK SMILES ON CENTENARIANS

Bob was celebrating his one-hundredth birthday at the senior home. Dozens of people were in attendance, including his children, grandchildren, and great-grandchildren.

Bob had been sent across the ocean at age twelve to escape the war in Europe. He lived in a succession of abusive foster homes until he was old enough to fend for himself. Bob never returned to his home country. He worked hard to succeed despite many challenges and setbacks, including the untimely death of his wife.

When Bob was asked what he attributed his longevity to, he said: "Here's the secret. Every morning when you wake up, the very first thing you do is: smile. Look out the window. If it's a beautiful day, sun shining: smile. If it's pouring rain, smile even wider—the farmers will be happy because it means a better crop! Every day when I wake up, I look for a reason to smile. Smiling leads to happiness. Happiness makes you healthy. That is my secret to long life."

Laughter has many specific health benefits. Research has found that laughter boosts the immune system by increasing levels of natural killer cells. It reduces the stress hormone cortisol and has an analgesic effect on chronic pain. Laughter exerts an antidepressant effect by increasing serotonin and dopamine levels in the brain.

It has positive physical effects such as improved breathing and relaxing muscles. It lowers blood sugar levels, improves relaxation, and even leads to beneficial bacterial changes in the intestinal system. It helps counter heart disease both through stress reduction and improved arterial blood flow. It has been identified as an effective therapy in a number of conditions: arthritis, allergies, eczema, diabetes, bronchitis. Laughter is good for you.

However, laughter was not Bob's secret to a long, healthy life. Bob was referring to finding a reason to smile each day. Bob was not a person who laughed a lot. He was a person who was able to find a reason to smile and be positive about things on a daily basis, no matter how difficult the circumstance in which he found himself. Bob's philosophy of smiling means to live life from the standpoint of gratitude.

In my line of work, I see how one's attitude and perspective toward an illness can greatly influence the outcome, both positively and negatively. Consider the following case studies, Richard and Sam, two men who approached a serious health issue from very different perspectives.

A TALE OF TWO PERCEPTIONS

Richard was a forty-five-year-old man with three young children, although the demands of his high-powered executive job meant he was largely an absentee parent. Richard suffered a massive myocardial infarction (heart attack). A coronary angiogram showed left main and severe three-vessel disease, and he was rushed to bypass surgery.

During the post-surgery years, he repeatedly expressed gratitude for the heart attack that gave him back his life. Although he still has the same stressful and demanding executive job, his approach and reactions have dramatically changed. He now finds joy and enthusiasm from coaching his sons' sports teams.

A weight has been lifted from him and he feels younger and healthier than he did before his surgery. He now laughs off situations that would have distressed him previously, instead focusing his thoughts on his children's laughter and their smiling faces, and always being grateful.

Sam, in contrast, reacted to his heart attack and coronary intervention with an attitude of distress and a feeling of unfairness. He felt he had been practicing healthy habits and was angry at being disadvantaged by his family history.

His father had died in his late sixties and Sam believed he, too, was doomed to a short life span. He was displeased and in despair at being unable to control events in his life. Sam fit the type A personality description, and his wife said he did not know how to relax and enjoy life.

Within a year, Sam's negative outlook was fulfilled when he had a second heart attack. Still, he persists with his disparaging and negative outlook toward life, and neither his wife nor I has been able to convince him of the need to change.

Although a change in attitude is not the only factor impacting improved health for Richard, he adopted a positive perspective that has allowed him to find enjoyment in each day of life. He is thankful for his health and the good things in life, regardless of what the future may hold. Sam, on the other hand, continues to see only the negative, and in expecting an early death, he may well find prophetic fulfillment.

Finding a reason to smile is not an artificial, glass-half-full perspective. It is not always easy to find a positive in every negative or a silver lining in every cloud. There are times where life throws us so many challenges, one on top of another, that you may wonder, "Can things get any worse?"

I urge you to suspend the natural instinct to be negative or immediately let your thoughts go to worry or fear, and allow yourself time and space to see what possible good there may be in this occurrence.

Humor and negative emotion cannot dwell within the same psychological space.

It is possible to reframe your thinking to find something in every turn of life that you can feel grateful for. Finding a reason to smile each day means cultivating a positive outlook and finding something good to celebrate when we wake up each morning. If we start out each day with a smile and a feeling of gratitude, we are motivated to see each experience from that perspective.

Adjust your expectations toward the positive and you are more likely to find reasons to smile. As you find more reasons to smile, you will bring the healing power of laughter into your life as well.

I want to share a prayer taught to me by my mentor Mary Morrissey. It comes from the Seicho-No-Ie or Truth of Life Movement in Japan:

SPIRIT OF JOY

INDWELLING ME

EVER PRESENT

I CALL YOU FORTH NOW

We can choose to be happy and laugh, or else we can laugh to be happy. One psychologist expressed it this way: humor and negative emotion cannot dwell within the same psychological space. If you always have humor in your life, unhappy and distressing emotions are less likely to find room within your heart. Finding a reason to smile each day may not always be easy, but the health benefits it will bring make it worthwhile.

R E N E W A B L E   E N E R G Y   F O R   T H E   H E A R T

L I V I N G   I N   T H E   F A S T   L A N E

Kate suffered from profound depression about twenty years ago, which almost cost her her life. She fought back and worked hard to regain her mental health. Knowing the symptoms of depression and being very familiar with the triggers, Kate always monitored her health and mental well-being. She returned to university, became a regular community volunteer, and took an active role in helping parent her grandchildren.

Unable to find work in her chosen field, she compensated by working three jobs. Kate had not taken a vacation in many years, but she hoped that her hard work would eventually pay off and that she could enjoy a break. She loved to play piano and had been a professional musician, but she hadn't played in years. She also loved writing and had plans to write a book one day when she finally found time.

Even though she had occasional chest pains, Kate watched her diet, spent quality time with her grandchildren, and tried to keep a positive outlook.

At the age of fifty, life was starting to beat Kate down. She suffered an unexpected financial setback and was suddenly faced with losing her home of thirty years to foreclosure. In quick succession, three members of her family died unexpectedly—one from cancer, two from heart attacks. Kate was then advised that due to cutbacks at her company, she was being laid off.

Kate thought she was contending with difficulties, but one day she awoke too sick to get out of bed. Her illness dragged on for several weeks. She soon found herself losing motivation and unable to concentrate on anything. One day, with horror, Kate realized that she had slipped back into full-blown depression.

Kate thought she was doing the right things, taking care of her health, always demonstrating a positive perspective, treasuring the good things in life, yet she was too caught up in the daily events of life. She was living at high speed, using stress as fuel, and not taking care of herself.

Although an accomplished musician, Kate had no time to play piano, nor did she have time for the things that nurtured her emotional health. Her focus was on working, helping her children, and raising her grandchildren. She had no time for friends or for herself, and she simply obscured her loneliness with other activities.

Kate fell victim to the negative effects of fight-or-flight syndrome—the acute stress response. She did not build long-term energy reserves and became accustomed to reliance on adrenaline and stress for fuel. Her immune system was the first to go, and once her body had become depleted of the deep energy reserves needed for sustenance, she fell victim to depression.

Life passes us by so quickly that we don't have time to stop and savor the moment. Yet, as Kate discovered the hard way, if we live under the sustained stress of a fast-paced life for any ongoing length of time, at some point our body is going to rebel and force us to slow down. Why not instead make a conscious effort to slow down the pace before that happens and before irreversible damage is done to your body?

The very act of slowing down and embracing the moment will help conserve valuable energy. It will allow your body to regenerate and renew.

It will create a receptive environment whereby you can start to build sustainable and renewable energy within. When you slow down the pace, you will be able to find time for creative pursuits—the art, music, and dance that will nurture your spirit and energize your emotional heart.

M I N D - B O D Y   A X I S

SLOWING DOWN THE PACE

Here are ten deliberate choices you can make to help you slow down and start using sustainable energy to power your life:

1. **Do less.** Make an assessment of what is really important and necessary. Focus on what needs to be done, and let go of the rest. Don't be afraid to leave unscheduled gaps in your day.

2. **Focus on the present**, not what you need to do tomorrow or what happened yesterday. Don't let the outside world distract you from what you are doing.

3. **Disconnect.** Unplug your iPhone or Blackberry, and shut off your laptop. A constant stream of incoming information keeps us in a constant state of stress and readiness.

4. **Appreciate nature.** Go outside, breathe fresh air, and enjoy the greenery. Take a nature walk. Feel the sensations of water and wind and earth against your skin. Listen to the birds.

5. **Do everything more slowly.** Eat slowly and savor each bite. Don't rush when driving to your next destination.

6. **Find pleasure in everything.** Instead of griping about washing dirty dishes, observe the lovely rainbow made by the soap bubbles. Sing while you scrub. Embrace your joie de vivre.

7. **Reconnect with life.** Make an unplanned visit to someone you love. Visit the zoo and marvel at the animals. Watch an ant on the sidewalk. Press some autumn leaves.

8. **Breathe.** When things get hectic, when stress starts to fuel you, take a deep breath. Become aware of your body and your breathing. Count. Listen to your heartbeat with each breath.

9. **Do something nice for someone.** The act of being kind takes time and forces you to slow down.

10. **Spend a little time with yourself.** Sit down and complete a crossword puzzle, or play a tune on your guitar. Do an intensive workout or simply listen to your heartbeat.

CHAPTER 7

REINVIGORATE YOUR MIND

"Tension is who you think you should be. Relaxation is who you are."
—Chinese Proverb

If you are like most people, you have experienced stress and anxiety at some point in your life. Not only does stress create unpleasant feelings, it can manifest in physical symptoms that include headaches, dizziness, difficulty sleeping, sweaty palms, loss of appetite, indigestion, and muscle tension. What you may not realize is that when you are stressed, your chances of having a heart attack, stroke, or coronary episode are also greatly increased.

Although stress may be caused by external factors that are often outside our control, there are ways to manage how we respond to stress. Western medicine tends to overlook the complex connections between mind and body, but when your mind is not at peace, the physical body is also disrupted. A healthy heart cannot exist without a healthy mind.

A healthy heart cannot exist without a healthy mind. Looking after your mental and emotional health is just as important as taking care of your physical health.

Looking after your mental and emotional health is just as important as taking care of your physical health.

How Can I Battle Stress?

"The greatest weapon against stress is our ability to choose one thought over another."

—William James

Most of my patients understand the importance of reducing stress in their lives, but many are not aware of how to do it. A demanding career, the loss of a loved one, financial difficulties, and health problems can all lead to a dangerous level of stress hormones in the body, yet all these events are largely outside of our control. These sources of stress are part of daily living, so we must learn ways to handle stress and overcome the negative emotions and destructive physical effects that come along with it.

It is important to recognize the symptoms of stress, including depression and anxiety. Fortunately, there are many ways to overcome the negative effects of stress in our lives. Eating well, exercising, resting, and avoiding high-stress situations are a good start. In addition, practices such as mindfulness, meditation, hypnosis, and vibrational healing can drastically improve mental well-being, reinforcing your mental ability to handle stress and reinvigorating the mind and heart.

Controlled Breathing

When something upsets you, take a deep breath. Controlled breathing, the simple action of taking deep, measured breaths, is a very effective way to manage stress on the spot. It can significantly reduce your blood pressure, regulate your heart rate, and prevent your body from releasing stress hormones. In addition, deep breathing promotes good circulation by introducing vital oxygen into the bloodstream. I like to do controlled breathing even when I am not particularly stressed, as I find it is an excellent way to relax and focus the mind.

Controlled breathing is incredibly easy to practice, as it is something your body does naturally. That being said, most people only use a fraction of their lung capacity when they breathe. To get the most out of your lungs' capacity, sit or stand in a comfortable position and breathe in deeply and slowly through the nose. Your lungs should fill up completely, and the lower part of your stomach should rise (abdominal breathing). Hold the breath for a second, and then slowly exhale through your mouth. Repeat this a number of times until you feel relaxed and calm. If you start to feel lightheaded, stop and continue normal breathing.

The next time you feel stressed, take a few deep breaths. You may be surprised at just how quickly the stress dissipates, and how reenergized you feel.

MEDITATION

Meditation is one of the most beneficial things you can do for mind and body. Not only does it relieve stress and reduce levels of adrenaline and cortisol, but studies show that meditation activates disease-fighting genes in your body.

Harvard Medical School researchers studied the genetic profiles of people who regularly meditated and practiced yoga. They discovered the presence of several active genes that were capable of fighting off heart disease, diabetes, inflammation, hypertension, and cancer. These genes were not as active in people who did not practice relaxation techniques; however, when these people began to meditate regularly, their genetic profiles became similar to those who regularly practiced yoga and meditation.

Even ten minutes of daily meditation will allow a brief, rejuvenating escape from a busy lifestyle filled with work obligations, family responsibilities, commuting, errands, chores, and paying bills. Meditation can hone your thought processes so that you have a clearer picture of what is truly important to you. You can meditate at home, at the office, on vacation, or while walking along the beach or through your neighborhood. Meditation costs nothing, but the rewards you reap are priceless.

After dabbling in meditation for several years, I finally made a full commitment to the practice. The difference I noticed was staggering. While meditation of any length and frequency will confer results, to truly experience its full benefits, you need to integrate the practice into your daily routine as an essential component of your life that is not to be sacrificed— much in the same way we consider sleep or meals to be indispensable. I believe that our personal commitment regarding things like this creates an energetic shift to which the universe responds.

Personally, my visit to Sedona in Arizona was an example of this response. My family had planned our spring break vacation to the Grand Canyon one year in advance. At the time, I knew nothing of this hidden, sacred land called Sedona. Then, two months into my dedicated meditation practice, I visited a Dahn yoga facility and there was a poster of Master Ilchi Lee's book, *The Call of Sedona*, hanging on the wall.

The majestic image of the deep red rocks against the crystal-blue sky immediately caught my attention. I soon learned that the Native Americans call Sedona "the land where Mother Earth's energy, which gives eternal life, comes out." Later, when we embarked on our vacation, I felt blessed to be able to stand on this magnificent land, to climb among the energy vortexes of Bell Rock and Cathedral Rock, and to watch the breathtaking sunset as I connected with Mother Earth, myself, and my family.

Mindfulness Meditation

When was the last time you took a deep breath, looked around, and were completely aware of what was happening at that very moment? If you are like most people, you probably cannot remember the last time you focused on the present.

As highly intelligent beings, we can simultaneously think about the past, present, and future. Unfortunately, this mental multitasking can lead us to dwell in the past, stress over what happened yesterday, or worry about what will happen tomorrow or one week or one year from now. We forget to simply enjoy what is right here in front of us. This is where mindfulness comes in. It allows us to appreciate the present rather than spending our time stressing over things that are beyond our control.

The concept of mindfulness is central to Buddhism; however, people of all religions, cultures, ages, and backgrounds can benefit from this practice. Many Western psychologists now use the concept of mindfulness to treat mental conditions such as anxiety and depression. Research has shown that it boosts the immune system and is effective in reducing feelings of loneliness that present a risk factor for cardiovascular disease in older adults.

Mindfulness means being aware of the body and mind at any given moment. It involves focusing on the present and concentrating on your breath and bodily functions, your thoughts, emotions, and physical surroundings. Some simple mindfulness exercises include conscious breathing, walking meditation or sitting meditation, and focusing on an object of awareness to pull you back into the present.

Transcendental Meditation

"Through Transcendental Meditation, the human brain can experience that level of intelligence which is an ocean of all knowledge, energy, intelligence, and bliss."

—Maharishi Mahesh Yogi

Transcendental Meditation (TM) is different from other forms of meditation because it focuses strictly on the mind, without interference from thoughts of breathing or other physical exercises. I make it a point to practice TM on a regular basis, because it helps me to manage stress more efficiently, settles my mind, helps me to think more clearly, and just makes me feel more relaxed and at peace.

TM is very easy to do. All you need is a comfortable place to sit with your eyes closed. The practice involves focusing on a sound or silently repeating a mantra to allow the mind to settle inward so that you feel rested and calm, yet are still deeply aware of your body, your thoughts, and your surroundings. This is done for twenty minutes, two times a day, to decrease stress, improve mental clarity, and encourage peace of mind.

Many studies on TM suggest that the practice can help to dilate blood vessels, decrease stress hormones, lower the heart rate, and encourage good cardiovascular health. A study at the Medical College of Wisconsin that was funded by the National Heart, Lung, and Blood Institute showed that people who practiced TM on a regular basis saw a 47 percent decrease in heart attacks, strokes, and deaths when compared to people who did not meditate.

TM is an excellent way to reinvigorate the mind and improve your cardiovascular health at the same time.

Guided Meditation

Another practice that I enjoy is guided meditation. It is very easy to do and promotes better health for the mind and the body. It is also an effective tool for gaining self-insight. Guided meditation can be great for beginners because you can walk through the process step by step with a teacher in a class or with an audio CD.

To practice guided meditation, you simply sit in a comfortable position, relax the muscles, and focus on breathing deeply. The teacher or CD will encourage you to visualize a specific situation or image. This could be anything from a beautiful setting, a positive energy entering the body as light or water, or a scene or image of your choice.

Visualization is incredibly empowering because it allows you to use your imagination to create your own reality. In this way, you are actively creating what you want in life, whether it be better health, more meaningful relationships, or increased happiness.

Chakra Meditation

Chak-ra (noun): any of several points of physical or spiritual energy in the human body, according to yoga philosophy. In Hinduism there are seven and in Tantra there are four major chakras.

—Merriam-Webster Collegiate Dictionary

Asian cultures have been aware for centuries that the body has a life force that cannot be seen by the naked eye. Ayurvedic medicine and traditional Chinese medicine focus centrally on this life force to keep body and mind healthy and happy. As a doctor with knowledge of both Western and Eastern practices, I do not doubt the existence of an invisible source of energy within us that needs to be kept in balance for optimum health. One way to keep this energy flowing is by balancing the chakras.

Chakras are central points in the body that channel energy, support the vital organs, and balance the physical, mental, and emotional states in the body. The common belief is that there are seven main chakras that run from the top of the head down to the base of the spine (see discussion in chapter 1). Chakra meditation allows you to concentrate on these vital points to improve energy flow, revitalize your physical body, and increase mental clarity.

To practice chakra meditation, start by sitting in a comfortable position and breathing deeply to relax the body. Try to calm the mind and concentrate on your core, the very center of your body.

Once you find your center, start with the chakra at the base of your spine and imagine energy flowing into the chakra and then spreading throughout the body. This can be achieved by visualizing light, water, or heat spinning outward from the chakra. After a few minutes, move on to the sacral chakra and repeat the process. Gradually make your way up through the solar plexus, heart, throat, and brow chakras, ending with the chakra at the crown of the head.

After a chakra meditation session, you should feel more energetic, grounded, and connected to your body.

Loving Kindness Meditation

Loving kindness meditation is an ancient practice steeped in Buddha's teachings. The Dhammapada, a collection of Buddha's quotes, contains this saying: "Hatred cannot coexist with loving-kindness, and dissipates if supplanted with thoughts based on loving-kindness." This form of meditation is geared toward achieving a gentle and systematic shift in thinking patterns. It is meant to transition the practitioner from a state of negative low-energy vibration to one of positive high-energy vibration.

Loving kindness meditation can be practiced in a seated position or it can be combined with walking. Gently focus your mind and visualize your breath as a shining, warm ray of light and love. This ray is first directed inward toward yourself, radiating through the heart and body. From there, you begin to direct it outward, initially toward a loved one, then toward a person of neutrality, and finally toward a person of hostility. Blessings of happiness, peace, love, forgiveness, and freedom from suffering should be bestowed on yourself and others during the visualization.

Barbara Fredrickson, Professor of Psychology at the University of North Carolina, demonstrated in her research lab that loving kindness meditation is an effective technique to generate positive emotions toward self and others. This type of meditation not only strengthens social connectivity, but also directly modulates the vagus nerve, thereby improving cardiovascular and whole-body physical health.

HYPNOSIS AND HYPNOTHERAPY

Some of my patients try meditation and mindfulness exercises, but they just cannot seem to shake the stress and anxiety that has built up inside them over the years. After reassuring them that this is very common for many people, I suggest that they consider hypnotherapy.

Now, the first reaction is often one of disbelief or humor. "You mean a guy dangling a watch in front of my face while chanting 'you are getting sleepy'?" Or they envision a group of people acting ridiculous on stage, following the hypnotist's instructions for the amusement of the audience. Some even think hypnotism is dangerous, having read novels about hypnotists who plant deadly posthypnotic suggestions and control people without their knowledge.

When it comes to hypnotherapy, however, nothing could be further from the truth. Hypnotherapy uses the mind-body connection to effectively bypass the waking mind and directly influence the nervous system in ways not possible during ordinary conscious states.

With hypnotherapy, you can access a natural state of heightened and focused attention that allows you to focus your thoughts, block out external stimuli, and concentrate on one particular thing at a time. Hypnotherapy can help you deal directly with mental, emotional, and physical problems such as stress, anxiety, fear, depression, guilt, pain, or addiction.

In a typical hypnotherapy session, you will discuss the problems you want to tackle with a certified hypnotherapist, who is a trained and competent health-care professional. People are often not aware of the root of their problems and simply want help diagnosing the symptoms. The hypnotherapist will ensure that you are comfortable and have you do some exercises to help focus the mind. These can include concentrating on breathing, repeating phrases to relax the body and mind, or using visualization.

Once you have reached a meditative state and entered a deeper level of awareness, the hypnotherapist may ask questions to focus on the problem and suggest ways that you can tackle the issues that are causing you distress or pain. Throughout the entire session, you are in complete control of your thoughts and actions.

Experts believe that hypnosis works on many levels to improve health and overall well-being.

- Hypnotherapy helps calm the body and focus the mind, which can lower blood pressure and decrease stress.

- A hypnotherapy session allows you to explore the subconscious, promoting greater self-awareness and the ability to control negative emotions and thoughts.

- While in a hypnotic or meditative state, you may be more open to suggestions and have an enhanced understanding of how to make positive changes in your life.

Studies also show that hypnosis can help reprogram the brain so that you experience positive physiological responses to certain stimuli rather than negative reactions such as fear, anxiety, and depression. This makes hypnotherapy a particularly efficient treatment for people suffering from trauma, phobias, addictions, or anxiety attacks.

EMOTIONAL FREEDOM THERAPY (EFT) OR TAPPING

Imagine if I told you that you could reprogram your mind to feel more confident, to be less anxious and stressed, and to be able to accomplish anything you set your mind to—just by using the power of your own mind and your fingertips.

When I first heard of Emotional Freedom Therapy (EFT), or tapping, I was a bit skeptical. I thought that there was no way simply tapping certain points on the body and repeating a phrase could change the way you think to reduce stress and pain and to increase confidence and motivation. However, psychological studies and scientific research suggest that this simple practice can have positive effects on the mind and body.

TAPPING STRESS AWAY

Ellen, a retired television producer, was sixty-nine years old and had been having chest pains for six months when she came to see me in December 2012. Although the chest pains had been the original reason for her visit, I soon learned that Ellen suffered from other conditions as well, including anxiety, insomnia, and two forms of acid reflux disease.

Ellen's anxiety was so bad that it was causing her joint and muscle pain, and her insomnia was debilitating to the point where she had been on prescription sleeping pills for ten years. An echo-cardiogram and an EKG revealed that her heart was fine. However, given her other ailments, Ellen opted to put her name on the list for my wellness center's newsletter.

The first one she received contained an invitation to Nick Ortner's online Tapping World Summit. Skeptical at first, Ellen joined the summit and ventured an experiment with tapping. Immediately, she experienced relief from her anxiety. After a few more sessions, her chest, muscle, and joint pains were greatly reduced. Three months later, Ellen was continuing to improve on her remaining symptoms with her tapping practice in conjunction with acupuncture.

Today, Ellen's chest pain is 95 percent gone, her acid reflux symptoms have diminished by 65 percent, her anxiety has been reduced by half, she is off of her prescription sleeping pills, and her muscle and joint pain has been completely eradicated.

EFT works on the same basic concept as acupuncture. According to traditional Chinese medicine, there are meridians in the body that transfer energy, or qi, to vital organs such as the brain or heart. Sometimes these meridians can become blocked, which results in poor health. Acupuncture points stimulate the energy flow through the meridians to restore a healthy balance.

Tapping involves focusing on a problem in your life and creating a phrase that acknowledges the problem while accepting who you are despite this problem. As you repeat the phrase, you tap on key points on the body to eliminate emotional blockages. Tapping stimulates the meridians in the same way acupuncture does, allowing positive energy to flow through the body. Unlike acupuncture, however, tapping is easily accessible and can be practiced anywhere and anytime using nothing more than your fingertips and your thoughts.

There are nine tapping points located on our heads and upper bodies, as Figure 7-1 suggests. Simply tap lightly on each of these areas while stating a truth about how you feel followed by a positive affirmation.

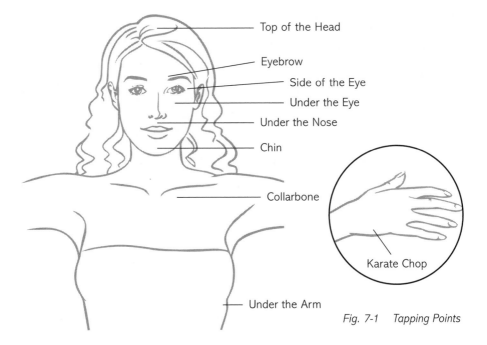

Top of the Head

Eyebrow

Side of the Eye

Under the Eye

Under the Nose

Chin

Collarbone

Karate Chop

Under the Arm

Fig. 7-1   Tapping Points

The sequence that I use is the karate-chop point, the eyebrow, the side of the eye, under the eye, under the nose, the chin point, the collarbone area, under the arm, and finally the top of the head. Repeat this cycle as many times as you feel necessary until there is an improvement in your emotional state or in your pain level.

 Nick Ortner's book *The Tapping Solution* is an excellent resource for those who wish to investigate the potential of tapping in greater depth. You can also refer to his website, www.yourvibrantheart.com/thetappingsolution, for more details on this practice.

Science has proven that EFT can have powerful effects on the brain, stimulating a part of it called the amygdala. The amygdala is responsible for creating the threat response, which is why we feel fear, anxiety, and aggression when we recall certain traumatic or stressful thoughts. This area of the brain is activated during post-traumatic stress reaction. We can reproduce the same biochemical response in the amygdala by repeating a phrase that brings a stressful situation to mind.

By simultaneously tapping specific areas on the body while repeating the phrase, signals are sent to the amygdala to stop producing the threat response, and you become less stressed about specific problems. EFT helps to reprogram the brain through a process called neuroplasticity, which rewires the neural connections in the brain. The power of EFT is now being used by psychologists to help treat trauma, addictions, physical pain and illness, phobias, anxiety, and stress.

A HEALING CALMNESS

Mary is forty-five. For almost two decades she has been dealing with heart palpitation episodes, and she has learned to link their occurrence with her stress levels. However, the episodes have been increasing in severity and intensity, becoming more unpredictable over the past few years.

Previously she would experience palpitations once every three months, but they are now occurring twice a week, sometimes daily. Mary's life circumstances seem closely linked with this increase in frequency and unpredictability. In addition, two of her children will soon be leaving her household to serve in the military.

I introduced Mary to tapping and was pleased to hear that she has been working with a healer to explore different types of emotional freedom release, meditation, and hypnosis. Mary strongly believes that her life has become settled as a result of these practices.

Were it not for these healing modalities, there is no question in my mind that Mary would have needed cardiac medications to control arrhythmia. She believes she can continue to avoid medication and instead manage her tremendous stress through her work with the healer. I'm inclined to agree.

Tapping is the modality that I personally use the most. I love its ease and simplicity, not to mention its speed and efficacy in producing the desired results. Not only do I recommend this method to all my patients to deal with the stress and anxiety of daily living and to help manage things like hypertension, chest discomfort, and palpitation, but I also consider it an invaluable tool that parents can teach their children to help the latter achieve their maximum potential.

For example, I love to share this story about my eldest son, Jonathan. One day, Jonathan was outside practicing his shots before a basketball game. I watched him brick about twenty attempts, becoming increasingly frustrated with every miss. So I asked him to stop shooting for a moment, and to start tapping. As you would expect from any twelve-year-old, there was some resistance. Eventually, my persistence won the day in the end. Jonathan did his tapping, which calmed him right away. He then went on to swish his next ten shots, including several three-point baskets. Tapping had cleared the mental blocks that were impeding his maximum potential. I also recommend tapping as a method to help upset children settle down to sleep.

BRAINWAVE ENTRAINMENT

Our amazing and complex brain is driven by electrical waves that vibrate at different frequencies. The speed of these frequencies determines our state of awareness, from deep sleep to high alertness, causing our heartbeat to slow or speed up accordingly. What if we could harness the velocity of these waves and alter the frequencies at will? Would it be possible to control how alert or calm we felt to better manage our mental and emotional state? Many scientists believe the answer is yes.

To understand the possibilities, we must first understand how brain waves work. All sound frequencies produce unique waves, measured in Hertz (Hz). The brain generates several different frequencies. Faster vibrations make us more alert, while the slowest vibrations occur during deep, dreamless sleep.

Our bodies access natural regenerative and healing processes when we are in the deepest sleep stages. Profound relaxation also rejuvenates and energizes us. When we experience stress over an extended period, the brain enters a heightened state of readiness. As we've learned, this stressful fight-or-flight response causes a chemical reaction that is extremely damaging mentally, emotionally, and physically, leaving us vulnerable to emotional and physical illness. To heal our mind and body, we need our brain to generate low-frequency waves and enter a deep relaxation state.

We can enter that state of profound, healing relaxation through meditation methods or hypnotherapy. We can also access relaxation by controlling the frequency of brain waves, using brain entrainment. Entrainment evokes the EEG (electroencephalographic) frequency-following response in the brain.

This can be illustrated with tuning forks. If a tuning fork is struck and begins to vibrate at 440 Hz, when brought near another tuning fork, the second will also begin to vibrate at 440 Hz. The same powerful response occurs in the brain. If a regular and consistent rhythmic stimulus is presented, the brain will respond by synchronizing its own electrical waves to match the rhythm.

A method of brain frequency entrainment being researched is binaural beats. This is an effect created when two audio tones of slightly different pitches are heard by right and left ears simultaneously. Similar to the tuning fork phenomenon, the brain responds by altering wave patterns to become entrained to a new frequency. By listening to the right binaural beat, listeners can slow down the frequency of their brain waves into a natural meditative state, where the brain can access the body's regenerative powers.

Research into binaural beats and brain entrainment as a therapeutic technique shows promise. There are commercial recordings of binaural beats available, but open-source software also makes it possible to record your own. You can obtain a free sample of a meditation track using this technology at www.yourvibrantheart.com/BWE.

VISUALIZATION

Visualization is the process by which we communicate our messages through the use of images, diagrams, and animations. Visualization allows us to access the subconscious mind nonverbally. As the saying goes, a picture is worth a thousand words. We can both reveal and express countless aspects of our inner selves through this process. During the process of creating art, our minds, emotions, and hearts become strongly interconnected, and often we create something unexpected that has been buried deep inside. Beyond the power of self-discovery, creative visualization can use this mind screen to create our new reality and affect or alter the exterior world or "our circumstances." We can, in essence, direct and produce the movie of our lives and script it to our hearts' desires.

Visualization is a powerful technique used by professional athletes, movie stars, successful business entrepreneurs, and others to improve performance. It can help overcome phobias, change behavioral patterns, and accelerate personal growth. By drawing on the principles of the Law of Attraction and positive visualization, we can begin to transform on a subconscious level the way we think. The Law of Attraction is backed by science and has proven to be a sustainable method for allowing the universe to bring the right people, places, and opportunities into our lives.

Vision boards use this powerful mind technology to employ positive thinking to first visualize and then achieve your dreams. Vision boards involve creating a large poster board filled with images that represent who you are and who you want to become.

Tangibles such as your desired job, where you want to live, and your ideal vacation all form part of the "big" picture. Various aspects of your health can be parts of the vision board: images of healthy, colorful fresh fruits and vegetables, fit bodies, young vibrant people enjoying life and participating in sports and activities, older people in prime health. While many people create these image boards manually, you can also build a virtual version on your computer using audiovisual representations, pictures, music, and word clouds.

Mind Movies offers such a technology and provides a visualization tool that empowers you to change your mindset and experience abundant success and happiness. The technology enables you to create your own personalized digital vision board with the uplifting images, powerful affirmations, and motivating music that you've chosen. Once you have created your vision board or mind movie, you can refer to it for inspiration and goal reinforcement.

I have been using Mind Movies since its initial launch and find it to be an easy and effective tool, especially for people who aim to make their dreams a reality (www.yourvibrantheart.com/mindmovies).

Regardless of which visualization format you prefer, the power comes from both the actual creation process, in which you learn about what things motivate you and why, and regular usage of your vision board for inspiration and reinforcement. It is not just the process but who we become in the process. Just as we grow and change, our vision board or mind movie is a living thing that will evolve with us over time as we gain new insights and achieve desired goals.

VIBRATIONAL ENERGY

Just as our brain operates on sound-wave frequencies, so does our physical body. Everything in this universe is made of atoms, each moving at a particular frequency. What distinguishes us from inanimate objects is the frequency at which we vibrate. Likewise, our physical body, our organs, our mental and emotional states, and our life-force energy all vibrate at specific and different frequencies. For optimum health, these frequencies must be kept in balance. What distinguishes a healthy person from an unhealthy person or a happy person from a sad person is the vibrational frequency at which our mind and body exist at that particular time.

Bruce Tainio of Tainio Technology in Cheney, Washington, showed that the ideal frequency for a healthy human body is between 62 and 68 MHz. If the frequencies dip below 62 MHz, the immune system is compromised, and illness and disease can set in.

Many factors can cause energy in the body to vibrate at a lower frequency, including pollutants, negative emotions (fear, anxiety, grief), stress, and past negative experiences. On the other hand, many things can raise the frequency, such as light, certain aromas, gentle touch and sounds, and feelings of love, joy, enthusiasm, and gratitude.

Vibrational healing, or energy healing, helps to correct imbalances in the vibrations in our bodies and brings harmony to our physical, mental, and emotional states. Acupuncture can clear energy blockages in the meridians of the body, as can tapping. Sounds, light, gems, aromas, flowers, or hands-on healing treatments all expose the body and mind to high-energy fields. These methods help heal the body, reduce negative emotions, and restore the body back to its natural frequency for optimum health.

A C U P U N C T U R E

C L E A R I N G   P A T H W A Y S   O F   P A I N

Ever since she was a teenager, Anita had experienced terrible migraines that started unexpectedly and lasted for hours. The pain was so severe that Anita felt nauseous and sometimes even

vomited. She was completely debilitated. With migraines occur-
ring every few weeks, all aspects of her life began to be seriously
affected.

I made several recommendations to help reduce Anita's pain
and stop the migraines, including changing her diet, exercising, and
meditating. Nothing, not even painkillers, seemed to help. Finally,
I recommended acupuncture. Although Anita was hesitant at first,
she eventually visited an acupuncture practitioner, who determined
that she was suffering from an imbalance brought on by emotional
stress. After just a few acupuncture sessions, Anita's pain was
gone. She now suffers migraines only about twice a year, at most.

Acupuncture is an ancient Chinese practice that has been used for centuries to correct imbalances in the body. Your body has pathways called
meridians, along which energy travels to nurture and support your vital
organs, tissues, and various systems. If meridians become blocked, there is
an imbalance in your qi, or life energy, and it cannot reach the places it is
supposed to go. When this happens, your body and mind become stressed
and ill.

These blockages can be removed by inserting tiny, thin needles into the
body at strategic points. In this way, acupuncture opens up the meridians,
restores energy, and promotes health and vitality. Acupuncture is used to
effectively treat a wide range of physical, mental, and emotional conditions, including pain, nausea, depression, addiction, and insomnia.

Many of my patients express apprehension and even fear at the thought
of being stuck full of needles. Although I understand their concerns, in
reality the experience is quite painless. Provided you choose an acupunc-
turist who has been certified by an official accrediting body, and one who

follows strict health and sanitation regulations, the experience should give you no cause for worry.

In a typical acupuncture session, the practitioner will ask you some questions about your symptoms and previous treatment. He or she will then check your pulse and your tongue to see where the problem lies. Once the problem has been identified, the practitioner will insert extremely thin needles into certain points on the body, just underneath the skin. Most people feel nothing, although they may experience a tingling sensation as the energy is activated in their bodies. The needles are left in for up to thirty minutes, and it usually takes only a few sessions to eradicate the problem.

Although acupuncture is most commonly used in the West to treat chronic pain, ongoing research into the treatment supports its efficacy for a number of medical issues. A recent study by the University of California, Los Angeles shows that acupuncture may be beneficial for patients who have experienced heart failure, as it suppresses the sympathetic nervous system, which can place pressure on the heart. It can improve circulation, decrease blood sugar, lower cholesterol, and effectively help with weight management.

AROMATHERAPY

Rich, fragrant flowers, newly cut grass, lush foliage—these smells represent the most pleasurable and invigorating aspect of a walk in the park. A particular aroma can bring a complete set of memories to vivid life. The sense of smell is powerful, connecting directly to our brain and our emotions. Smells can refresh us, enliven us, and make us feel at peace with the world and with ourselves. That is the central idea behind aromatherapy.

The ancient practice of aromatherapy involves taking the essence of plant materials and condensing them into oils, which are called essential oils.

Essential oils can be used by heating them and inhaling the aroma or by applying the oils directly to the body.

Each essential oil fragrance has a different effect on the body. For example, when I feel tired or run down, I often dab some peppermint or tea tree oil onto my wrists or temples for a quick boost of energy. If I feel stressed or anxious about something, a few drops of chamomile or rose oil in a diffuser help a great deal to calm my nerves.

Researchers believe that essential oils work in two ways to heal the body and promote good health:

- **Breathing in the scents.** This stimulates your brain to produce positive reactions for good physical, mental, and emotional health. Certain scents can reduce anxiety, stress, pain, depression, and nausea.

- **Absorbed by the skin.** Some essential oils have antibacterial and antimicrobial properties, and can strengthen the immune system. This makes them an effective tool for healing the body.

I discovered the truth of the latter when I cut myself on a tree branch while hiking. A good friend suggested applying lavender oil on the abrasion. Within hours the cut was less painful, the swelling had gone down, and it was already starting to heal. This natural and pleasant-smelling essential oil has been a staple in my medicine cabinet ever since.

Science shows that aromatherapy may also be good for your heart. A study at the Chiba University Graduate School of Medicine in Japan revealed that men who inhaled lavender oil showed significant decrease in the stress hormone cortisol, as well as improved coronary circulation. Other studies suggest that basil, thyme, and rosemary oils can help with circulation. Marjoram, rose, and peppermint contribute to improved heart strength; and lavender, marjoram, ylang ylang, and ginger can help in decreasing high blood pressure.

Furthermore, essential oils have vibrational frequencies of between 52 and 320 MHz, which can help to raise the energy levels in your body to reduce stress and fatigue, increase happiness, and fight off disease.

COLOR THERAPY

Have you ever wondered why red is such a common color on sale signs at your local supermarket? Why police uniforms are always blue or black?

Think for a minute about your favorite color, and imagine yourself wearing that color. How do you feel? Confident? Happy? Now think about your least favorite color and imagine wearing clothes in that color for an entire day. Now what do you feel? If you are like most people, your favorite color would make you feel comfortable and confident. The opposite would be true of a disliked color.

Colors have incredible power over our emotions and mental state. Color is created from the different frequencies of light energy, and different colors have varying electromagnetic energy fields and wavelengths. We are individually drawn to certain colors, perhaps because those colors fulfill a vibrational frequency in the body that is lacking. Color therapy is one way to correct such imbalances to make you feel more relaxed, happy, and at peace with yourself.

Color therapists use a number of tools and techniques to balance the energy in your body. A therapist may ask you to visualize a color that corresponds with a specific chakra to heal a certain area in the body. Colored gemstones, lamps that emit colored light, or monochromatic rooms may also be used to encourage the absorption of wavelengths emitted from a particular color.

Different colors are connected to different emotions, and each color affects the body and mind. For example, red can make your heart beat faster and encourage feelings of strength and ambition, while green can be very refreshing and calming.

While color therapists believe that certain colors can have profound effects on your mood, thoughts, and emotions, too much of one color can have the opposite effect. This is why it is a good idea to surround yourself with different colors on a regular basis.

COLOR	MEANING	BENEFITS	EXCESS/DETRIMENT
RED	energy, vitality, strength, courage, power, passion, aggression, sexual	overcome depression, self-confidence, security, power	aggression, anger, hostility, irritability, anxiety, stress
ORANGE	warm, joyful, social, happy, content, wisdom	inviting, optimistic, cheerful, inspiring	irritability, anxiety, agitation
YELLOW	intelligence, innovative, inspiration, optimism	clarity, focus, memory, empowerment, confidence	mental fatigue, exhaustion
GREEN	peace, hope, balance, self-control, harmony, love	calm, centered, stress reduction, relaxation	negative energy, laziness
BLUE	knowledge, creativity, decisiveness, harmony, sincerity	calm, peace, clarity, communication, relaxation	depression, insecurity, pessimism, fatigue
INDIGO	truth, intuition, imagination, understanding, serenity	intuition, awareness, perception, imagination, connection to spiritual self	depression, isolation
PURPLE	serenity, inspiration, faith, creativity	generosity, calm, artistic, altruistic	depression, insecurity, negative emotions
LAVENDER	gentle, relaxing, awakening	balanced, centered, peace	tired, fatigue
WHITE	purity, innocent, optimistic	purify mind on the highest levels	—
SILVER	peace, persistence	removes diseases	—
GOLD	strength	strengthens the body and spirit	too strong for many people
BLACK	silence, elegant, powerful	silence and peace	aloof, intimidating
GREY	stability	inspires creativity and symbolizes success	—

Fig. 7-2   Color Chart

CRYSTAL HEALING

Crystals and gemstones hold a fascination and are highly appealing. Children love to collect rocks, and adults enjoy wearing beautiful jewelry created from gemstones. They are much more than just pretty rocks, however. Some people believe that certain crystals and gemstones have the power to carry high-frequency energy to our bodies to help restore balance and promote good health.

Crystal healers use these stones as tools to rebalance and restore energy. A crystal healer will determine which of your chakras are in need of cleansing. Specific gemstones are then placed next to those chakras to harness the energy of the stones and heal the body naturally by raising the vibrational frequency. The energy of the crystals can make you feel lighter, more joyful, and invigorated. You can also wear healing crystals and gemstones as jewelry for an ongoing energy boost.

Many people say that they feel more relaxed when they have crystals placed next to their chakras. They are able to let go of negative feelings, attitudes, or habits that prevent them from getting the most out of life. Others report feeling energized and having an overall sense of well-being. Whether you believe in the power of crystals or not, enjoying their color and beauty will definitely brighten your mood.

INTEGRATED ENERGY THERAPY

Although many of us would love nothing more than to go through life encountering only positive experiences, that is not possible. We all suffer negative experiences at some point that cause us to feel guilt, fear, anger, and sadness. These experiences can strengthen us and help us to grow.

However, over time, negative energy can build in our cells, leaving imprints or marks that cause the vibrational frequency in the body to be imbalanced. This can lead to stress, depression, and poor physical health.

Integrated Energy Therapy (IET) is one way to cleanse the cells of these negative imprints so that you can eliminate the buildup of negativity, opening the mind and body to positive energy and allowing you to access your true potential. This can be a very enlightening and empowering experience.

In an Integrated Energy Therapy session, a certified practitioner will ask you to lie fully clothed on a massage table with your head on a pillow in a comfortable position. The practitioner will then use his or her hands to gently touch specific areas on the body that hold emotions and are susceptible to blockages. Sometimes relaxing music is used. The best thing about IET is that you do not need to resurrect negative past memories to rid yourself of these damaging emotions. Everything is released through the healing touch of the therapist.

Many people report feeling a great deal lighter after an IET session, and after a few sessions they begin to feel free from the limitations that held them back before. IET is an excellent way to balance the body and mind and become more connected with your true self, accessing your ability to create the life that you truly want.

LIGHT THERAPY

ANTIDOTE FOR THE BLUES

Robert is from New Hampshire, where winters can be long, cold, and dark. From a young age, Robert would go into deep depression every winter. He tried antidepressants, but he did not like the side effects. Eventually one of his therapists suggested that he add a bit more light in his life. Robert started escaping the winter by taking long trips to places like Florida, California, and Hawaii. Within days after arriving in these bright, sunny climates, his depression would lift.

When the recession hit, however, Robert could no longer afford the lengthy trips. Winter came, and depression returned. Robert began to look into different options. He discovered a light box that emitted 10,000 lux, which is similar to the light on a sunny day. When he used it, his sleep patterns improved, his mood lifted, and he felt more relaxed and healthier. It wasn't quite the same as a beach in Hawaii, but it was a close second!

Does your mood take a nosedive on gray, rainy days? You may be one of the 20 percent of people who suffer from seasonal affective disorder (SAD). This condition arises from a lack of natural light, and it can cause depression, insomnia, and fatigue. Even if you do not suffer from SAD, a long bout of dark and miserable days is enough to give anyone the blues.

One way to counteract this emotional reaction is with light therapy. By exposing your body to high-frequency light wavelengths, you can realign natural daily rhythms and elevate your mood. This reduces stress, depression, and other negative emotions that contribute to low-frequency energy vibrations in the body and poor health.

Scientists believe that light activates various physiological responses in the body. For example, when we are exposed to light on a daily basis, our body's internal clock is regulated. This photosensitive system is responsible for determining sleep patterns, maintaining body temperature, and releasing hormones that regulate moods.

Light is also a source of energy. When you are not getting enough light, your vibrational frequencies may drop, resulting in negative emotions and poor health. A study at the University Medical Center in Amsterdam found light therapy to be just as effective as, if not better than, antidepressants for people who suffered from SAD. Light therapy is a great alternative to synthetic drugs and an easy way to improve your mood and your health.

MUSIC AND SOUND THERAPY

Music is incredibly powerful. You hear a song and it lifts your spirit, makes you feel happy, energizes you, and gives you the feeling that you can take on the world. Songs can also evoke sadness and melancholy or bring on nostalgia and heartache. Music expresses emotions we may not be able to express in words.

It should therefore come as no surprise that music can be a very powerful tool for balancing our emotional, mental, and even physical states. Many cultures have been using music and sounds for centuries to increase the vibrational frequency of the body and mind and to promote good health. Today, psychologists and health-care professionals use music therapy to treat a wide range of conditions, including depression, anxiety, stress, insomnia, social disorders, and attention deficit disorder (ADD).

Not only can music reduce stress and elevate your mood, it may also protect your heart. In 2009, the Cochrane Heart Group researched twenty-three controlled trials that studied the effect of music on patients with coronary heart disease. They found that the patients who listened to music as part of their treatment had significantly reduced blood pressure and lower heart and respiratory rates than those who did not listen to music as part of their treatment.

Another study by the Johns Hopkins University revealed that stroke patients who listened to rhythmic music during rehabilitation were more flexible, felt happier, and enjoyed better-quality personal relationships than those who did not incorporate music into their rehabilitation.

There are many forms of musical therapy and many ways that you can use music to reinvigorate the mind and create a better quality of life. With Neurologic Music Therapy (NMT), a trained therapist studies the way your brain reacts to certain types of music and then develops a music plan to change the patterns in the way you think and your emotional responses.

Other music therapists use sounds with high-vibration frequencies—Tibetan bowls, didgeridoos, chanting, bells—to rebalance the energy flow in your body. In addition, there are many audio CDs and MP3s that are designed to create a deep state of relaxation and inner peace.

So the next time you find yourself feeling burnt out, stressed, or anxious, listen to some music. Let it refresh your mind, lift your mood, and rid you of any negative thoughts that are dragging you down.

REIKI

We've considered how negative emotions, stress, and low-frequency vibrations in the body can all lead to a deterioration in physical health. The good news is that the universe is full of positive energy that is free for the taking. Music, vibration, color, light, crystals—all provide ways to access this energy. Being able to channel the energy in a more directed way can help us reap huge physical and emotional rewards. This is where Reiki comes in.

Reiki is a way to harness positive energy to clear blockages and push out negative energy. Reiki practitioners are trained to find the physical locations that are causing mental, emotional, and physical stress. They draw on their ability and training to focus high-frequency, positive energy into these spots, encouraging the body to heal naturally and function more efficiently. Many people use Reiki to reduce pain and tension from injuries or stress, release negative emotions, or simply relax and promote well-being.

In a Reiki session, you sit or lie down on a table, fully clothed. The Reiki practitioner will assess the areas needing attention and then either gently touch these strategic locations or hover their palms a few inches from the body, holding position for a few minutes before moving on to the next location. You may feel slight warmth or a tingling sensation while the positive energy is being transferred into your meridians. A full session takes about an hour.

Although some people may scoff at Reiki, scientific studies indicate that it can have very positive effects on the cardiovascular system. In a 2010 study by the Yale-New Haven Hospital, patients with acute coronary syndrome saw significant decreases in heart-rate variability after Reiki was incorporated into their treatment programs.

In addition, a study at the South Glasgow University Hospital NHS Trust looked at the effects of Reiki on blood pressure, heart rate, and respiratory rate. Reiki was administered to one group of people, while the other group simply rested for thirty minutes. While both groups showed a decrease in heart and respiratory rates, only the Reiki group saw a significant decrease in diastolic blood pressure.

These studies suggest that Reiki can be a very powerful tool in the fight against cardiovascular disease.

REINVIGORATE YOUR MIND

We all know how important it is to care for our physical body, but few people take sufficient time to attend to the mind. When your mind is calm and at peace, you will find that you have increased energy, more motivation to accomplish your dreams, more confidence and creativity, and a higher quality of life. On the other hand, if you neglect your mental and emotional health, you may feel stressed, anxious, fearful, angry, or depressed. Moreover, these negative feelings are likely to be followed by physical ailments.

Your mind is one of your most important assets. If you treat it right, it has the power to help you achieve almost anything you could possibly dream of. So take care of your mind. Tend to your emotions and eliminate the negative thoughts that are holding you back. Your life will suddenly take on more meaning and purpose, and it will begin to resemble the life you truly want and deserve.

> Your mind is one of your most important assets. If you treat it right, it has the power to help you achieve almost anything you could possibly dream of.

CHAPTER 8

RESTORE YOUR SOUL

"As a well-spent day brings happy sleep, so life well used brings happy death."

—Leonardo da Vinci

Emotions have a profound effect on the soul. Regardless of the source, continual stress, daily cares, sadness, and grief all tear holes in our soul. All emotions, whether positive or negative, place stress on our heart, mind, and spirit. Unless we find ways to repair the damage, over time our souls become ragged and we start to lose touch with our core self. Our inner guide can lose definition and clarity. The power to direct our lives and make healthy choices is hampered. We begin to flounder and lose direction.

If you neglect your soul, it can wither away and become dormant. Your heart may continue to beat, but it no longer receives the vital spark of energy from the inner soul. Life no longer holds hope or promise, and your day-to-day existence becomes just that—existing.

You can, however, nourish your soul and restore it to health. The resurrection of your soul is a journey of exploration from within, in which you learn to listen to your subconscious and develop a strong relationship with your inner guide. Self-awareness is enhanced, and you become one with your spiritual self.

An examination of aspects of the core self relating to life and death is a good starting point for the soul-restoration journey. Death is an essential part of life, and our emotional perspectives on the topic can provide insight into ways to resurrect a damaged soul.

CONFRONTING DEATH

THE END-OF-LIFE STRUGGLE

The final six months of Ms. Levine's life brought the greatest sadness to my heart. Several heart attacks and severe strokes had left her body contorted, contracted, and fixed in a fetal position. Ms. Levine had suffered at least eight cardiac arrests, only to be successfully resuscitated each time. It seemed like every intern and resident in the hospital had had the opportunity to learn cardiopulmonary resuscitation on her.

Although each resuscitation kept Ms. Levine's heart pumping, and her respiratory system kept providing oxygenation to her blood cells, the multiple strokes and anoxic brain damage had rendered her nonverbal. I cared for her, yet never had the chance to truly know her or understand her deepest thoughts and wishes. Ms. Levine did not have a living will and had not expressed her wishes regarding life support before entering this state. Her nine children and grandchildren were left to make these decisions, and they could never reach consensus, so the resuscitation efforts continued.

The situation lasted for months. Cardiac arrest would be followed by successful resuscitation. The patient would be on an intubator and ventilator for several weeks, then extubated and moved to the regular ward, only to have another cardiac failure and end up back in the intensive care unit post-resuscitation.

She could not express her feelings, so I could only imagine what she must have been thinking as the interns and residents poked and prodded her in their dutiful attempts to save a life. I was the attending resident when she suffered her tenth cardiac arrest. Ms. Levine was not successfully resuscitated and was finally put to rest.

One of the most difficult situations we must experience is confronting death. Having been involved in four of the resuscitative efforts on Ms. Levine and having participated in many of the life-support discussions that the medical staff had with the family, I had a longitudinal perspective.

Given my Asian background and philosophy, my perspective on life and death is somewhat different from that of my colleagues. I firmly believe that decisions regarding life support and resuscitative efforts belong solely to the patient or to his or her surrogate, and while I firmly uphold the Hippocratic oath of supporting life and doing no wrong, I believe that we physicians are not obligated to offer all available medical intervention if these procedures and interventions are ultimately futile in restoring a life of quality. This is a difficult issue that transcends beyond medical practice to that of medical ethics.

While many of my colleagues struggle with having end-of-life discussions with patients and their families, I've never had those struggles. I view death as a beautiful part of life, a continuation onto another existence. When viewed from this perspective, death does not need to be feared or dreaded, but can be seen as a beautiful and even welcome transition, especially for someone who is suffering or who no longer has a good quality of life.

Often, we as physicians are unable to have independent and open discussions regarding the process of death due to our own fear of death. Instead, we place the burden on the patient or the family, who then must struggle with the guilt of making the critical decision of whether to resuscitate or choose death.

I frame this discussion from a different perspective. "Do not resuscitate" does not mean "do not care," since we continue to provide the best quality of care to their loved ones. In the event that the heart stops beating and lungs stop breathing, should all efforts be made to bring their loved ones back to life, given their current medical status? In the case of Ms. Levine, had the family taken the viewpoint that the afterlife would be better than the life their loved one was experiencing at the time, I believe the decisions regarding resuscitation might have been different.

Confronting the death of a loved one is difficult. No one wants to die. Even if you believe that heaven awaits, you don't want to die to get there. When we are put in the position of making a life-or-death decision for a loved one, our distress is compounded with guilt and other emotionally wrenching feelings.

Death, however, is a destination that awaits us all. If we can reframe that experience as a transition from a current life situation into another one, as a movement into a life that may be much better, the pain our heart experiences can be eased. The experience of death can also be used to celebrate life and serve as a way to reinforce and rejuvenate the soul, lifting the heart.

DEATH AND LIFE

ENERGIZING THE SOUL

A reception after a funeral is in progress. Profound sadness and condolences are being expressed in the social atmosphere. Hearts are heavy and everyone is seeking to find healing through shared remembrance. All at once, a crack of thunder introduces a rainstorm. The rain begins to pour down outside the reception hall.

Suddenly three small boys appear in the window. They have stripped off their shoes and socks and they are outside dancing in the rain in their formal funeral suits and vests. Their little faces are upturned to the sky, heedless of the water running down their chins and dripping off their shirts and ties. They are laughing ecstatically, caught up in the joy of the moment.

One by one, the adults are drawn to the window to watch. They begin to share sidelong, smiling glances at one another, half wishing they, too, could run out in the rain. The children's laughter becomes infectious, imbuing the sad gathering with an unexpected wash of sheer joy, an ecstatic embrace of one single moment of life.

What was it that allowed these children to embrace life in such a passionate and free way? To take such delight in a single, random moment? These little boys felt the sadness of the occasion. They, too, mourned the loss of a loved one, but for that moment they were able to let their emotions free and simply dance for joy in the rain, letting it cleanse them. They helped remind a roomful of adults that in spite of the profound sadness life sometimes brings, we can transcend the pain by taking hold of a single moment of life, celebrating it and enjoying it to the fullest.

As adults we sometimes forget how to find simple joy in that single moment of life. We have become preoccupied with worries, worn down by the stress of the day and the cares of tomorrow. We don't remember how to play, how to be young and free for a moment in time. Children, on the other hand, are invigorated by small things in life. They don't let cares and worries become a weight that slows them down and makes them tired. Rather than cower under an umbrella in a rainstorm, they embrace it and soak in its delights.

The act of embracing and celebrating a single moment of life lightens our hearts and lifts our spirits. It rejuvenates us physically and emotionally and restores our soul. A lesson can be learned from these small boys. Rather than allowing the cares of the day to continue to tear at your soul and spirit, become engaged in the joy of living for that moment. If it's raining, turn your face to the sky and taste it. Roll in the grass and squish your toes in the mud. Enjoy every sensation that comes with being alive.

There are a number of positive consequences to fully living and experiencing a single moment of life. An increased heart rate and improved circulation, an emotional uplift, a desire to smile for no particular reason, a letting go of weighty problems—these are all physical and emotional outcomes.

Even in the most difficult circumstances, we can extract a single moment that provides a reason to celebrate. As you connect with your inner self and enjoy that moment, your soul is energized with essential nourishment to counterbalance the negative emotions.

> Embracing and celebrating a single moment of life lightens our hearts and lifts our spirits.

If you are used to living life on adrenaline, fueled by stress, focusing on a single moment in time is not an easy thing to do. Slowing down the pace is an important first step, but one of the best ways to train yourself to focus and to find joy in a single moment is through meditation, in which you access a state of mind that is more receptive to your emotions and inner self.

Meditation puts you into a unique state of restful alertness, during which the sympathetic nervous system (the fight-or-flight response) is deactivated. The mechanisms activated during the stress response are effectively reversed, dilating blood vessels and reducing levels of stress hormones such as cortisol and adrenaline. Not only does this help reverse the harmful effects of stress, but this relaxed, meditative state provides a connection to your inner resources and creativity. Soul and spirit can then be nurtured with the help of your inner guide.

The right food, exercise, emotional nourishment, and lifestyle changes will rejuvenate your body, strengthen your heart, and revitalize your mind. However, gaining an understanding of our emotions and learning how to live soulfully and spiritually are also essential to heart health. To become empowered to choose the life you want, you need to connect with the inner self.

EMOTION AND THE SOUL

Emotions are an essential part of being human. They dictate our feelings and guide our actions. We learn emotional competence as a way to engage and function socially. Moods that are appropriate help us manage social situations and keep us safe. Fear ignites the fight-or-flight syndrome, while guilt and remorse can motivate apology and reparation. Anger can make us competitive and motivate us to act for change, and jealousy moves us to be protective. Curiosity sparks discovery, and pride motivates personal improvement. Expressing joy and happiness is contagious and inspires those around us, and love heals us and others.

We also use our emotions to express ourselves creatively. Powerful works of art and music have been born out of anger, love, despair, passion, hope, suffering, and ecstasy. We need to be able to express the complete spectrum of emotions, using them to manipulate our environment in good and bad ways.

However, emotions tax our soul. We've seen how sustained negative emotions can wear us down and leave us vulnerable to a host of physical ailments. Good stress can be equally as damaging as bad stress. Positive emotions can place a burden on us if we don't know how to manage them and find a balance. Too much sadness can harm the soul, but too much happiness can also be unhealthy.

A number of studies have shown that too much happiness can create psychological harm to our soul and spirit. This may seem counterintuitive to everything we have been saying so far, but in reality, one of the secrets to heart health is balance. Emotional balance is essential, and that means that in addition to finding ways to mitigate the effects of negative stress, we also must guard against falling into the dysfunctional realm of too much happiness.

How can excessive happiness harm our emotional soul?

First, the pursuit of happiness must not become an end in and of itself. If you only focus on the end result, you may not enjoy the journey along the way. You may also find that the outcome is not what you expected. For example, you may anticipate joy and happiness as you plan a wonderful fiftieth birthday party. Yet when the day arrives, you instead experience profound despair at the realization that your life is half over.

Intense happiness and emotional mood swings can impact our ability to channel inner creativity and make us less able to meet new challenges. The sense that we have achieved perfect happiness may create complacency and remove the desire to improve or to effect positive change on behalf of others.

An uninhibited happiness "high" can make us more prone to risk taking, perhaps making us inclined to eat or drink too much, under the excuse that we are happy and enjoying ourselves. If we only attend to the positives in our environment, we may not see signs of danger.

Traditional Chinese medicine and philosophy add support to the idea of a direct relationship between emotions and physical health. The concept of qi, or vital energy, perceives emotions as closely integrated with the organs. The heart is the source of all emotions and holds the essential spirit.

In three main Chinese philosophies—Daoism, Confucianism, and Buddhism—seven emotions are recognized. These are most commonly listed as: joy, anger, pensiveness/rumination, worry/anxiety, sadness/grief, fear, and fright/shock. Empathy is sometimes also included. The activity of each emotion is linked with injury to a specific organ, and because emotions originate in the heart, the heart will also sustain damage.

Normal emotional activity causes no disease or weakness, but when emotions cause excessive mental stimulation or become too powerful, they disturb the qi. This causes serious injury to the internal organs and leaves the body susceptible to disease. In these Chinese medicine philosophies, emotions also influence each other, and one emotion can control or mediate the negative effects of another. For example, grief controls anger, so angry feelings can be reduced by focusing on loss or sadness.

We've already considered the negative impact of emotions such as fear and grief, and most of us can understand the logical connection between the emotions and other physical harm. Although the presence of joy on the list may seem at odds with Western medicine, in reality the harmful joy that scatters the qi in Chinese tradition is a type of emotional excess linked with desire and craving. It has been compared to Western society's preoccupation with excitement and violence and the overstimulation of a fast-paced life, in contrast to peace and calm in the face of a storm.

Empathy is another emotion that is considered positive in Western tradition, yet can actually be harmful in excess. If we feel too much empathy, we can take on another's pain and disease, leaving us vulnerable and unable to remain objective. Professional health-care providers are aware of this danger and must monitor self-care and always be on guard to maintain healthy boundaries to avoid the risk of allowing feelings of empathy to contribute to personal stress.

Our physical health is damaged not only by extreme or excessive emotions, but also by suppressed emotions that we allow to build up inside. Both prolonged grief and unexpressed grief cause damage. Pent-up anger is just as harmful as constantly expressed rage. For these reasons, Western medicine recognizes the value of having healthy outlets for emotions such as anger and grief.

In each case, however, the key is understanding the link between emotions and health and finding a harmonious balance. For example, if we understand how joy in Chinese tradition causes injury to the heart by "scattering the spirit," we can counteract those effects by developing a calm and peaceful spirit to temper the joy.

A craving for fast-paced excitement can be potentially damaging if constantly indulged, so you can balance it with time spent appreciating the natural calm peace of a green garden. If you are a kind, empathetic person who is always helping others, you can find balance by building self-care, laughter, and music into your daily agenda.

Both negative and positive emotions are important to a grounded perspective that is emotionally healthy and well-balanced. Rather than simply seeking happiness, we should seek to learn how to create harmony between emotions, soul, and spirit. Even when we are presented with circumstances of emotional heartache, if we are connected with our inner emotional self, we will be able to manage those circumstances in a way that will not destroy or severely damage the soul, spirit, and heart.

FINDING YOUR INNER SPIRIT GUIDE

LISTENING TO THE LITTLE VOICE

Christine, a senior government executive and mother of two, had just celebrated her fiftieth birthday. Although she worked and lived in a high-stress environment, Christine paid attention to her diet and exercised regularly. Her health was relatively good, although she was overweight and her weight had become more difficult to control since quitting smoking several months before.

In the weeks leading up to her birthday, Christine had experienced occasional bouts of nausea and shortness of breath, but she put these down to seasonal flu and physical adjustments to quitting smoking. Sometimes Christine felt a vague premonition of doom, but she assumed that it was also related to anxiety and stress.

One afternoon, after engaging in a vigorous workout at the gym, Christine paused on her way home to help an elderly neighbor lift some heavy boxes from her car. Later that evening she began to feel pain and soreness in her upper back and arms, along with some pressure in the center of her chest.

Her first thought was that she had overexerted herself, but when she became flushed and clammy and started feeling a bit nauseous, a little voice inside suggested that something more serious might be happening. Christine did some Internet research, and verified that the symptoms were linked with heart attacks in women. A vague spark of memory prompted her to take an aspirin, just to be on the safe side. Christine made plans to visit her doctor in the morning.

The next day a stress test revealed a problem and the subsequent coronary angiogram provided the frightening news. Her left anterior descending artery (main artery to the front of the heart) was 99 percent blocked. Christine had suffered a heart condition known as the "widowmaker" because of its high mortality rate.

Profoundly shaken and grateful to be alive, Christine sent a message to friends and family reminding them to become familiar with the symptoms of heart attacks in women. She concluded with the comment, "The little voice inside is so easy to ignore. This time I listened to it, and it saved my life."

Many women with heart disease experience symptoms that are subtle and easily written off as nothing more than a flu or a response to stress or anxiety. Although chest pain and pressure is common, symptoms such as shortness of breath, nausea, and back or jaw pain are also common indicators of heart attack in women.

In many cases these symptoms can be experienced for some weeks before an attack. In the aftermath of a heart attack, many women report having felt a sense of dread or impending doom, but not having related it to their physical symptoms. In Christine's case, her physical body had been warning her, right up to the point when the voice inside prompted her to take her symptoms seriously.

The voice lives within all of us, and we have all likely sensed its presence. It is known as intuition and can serve as an inner guide to direct our decision making and help us attain greater self-knowledge. In some cases, it can save our life.

Our inner guide wears many forms and is understood and experienced in unique and individual ways. Some interpret it as intuition, an inner, all-knowing voice, a gut feeling that guides decision making, similar to one's conscience. It could be described as deep physical knowledge held within the subconscious below the general sense of awareness.

Many feel it as a powerful spiritual connection with a higher being. The inner guide may be the remembered counsel of a wise and respected grandparent that comes as a voice inside your head. It has been called the sixth sense or second sight, and it has been interpreted as premonition or clairvoyance.

At its most basic, the inner guide represents our connection to the person within. The connection is unique because the person inside each of us is multifaceted; a kaleidoscope of experiences, sensations, memories, hopes, motivations, and desires. On a conscious level we are not always aware of the elements that reside within, yet they are available if we know how to summon them.

When we access the inner guide, we gain self-knowledge and the ability to expand our conscious experience. Once we have developed a relationship with our inner advisor, we are able to draw on our intrinsic wisdom as needed.

To connect with your inner guide, start from a relaxed, meditative state, using visualization. Initially you may need to do this at a time when you are alone, with no external distractions. You can use meditative techniques, drumming, music, natural sounds—anything that helps you attain a state of complete relaxation and focus.

Ensure that every part of your body is relaxed, with no muscle tension to distract the process. Concentrate on what is going on inside your body and shut out all external stimuli. Listen to your breathing and experience the sound of your heartbeat and your breath. Then imagine a peaceful, restful place that can serve as a location where you can meet with your inner guide.

Once you have constructed the location in a comfortable receptive state, you can begin to visualize your inner self. Detailed instructions on how to establish and maintain a connection with your inner guide can be found in many places, and you can experiment until you find a method that suits your unique needs.

CONNECTING WITH YOUR INNER GUIDE

Making a connection to the guide within you is easier than you think. By simply slowing down and becoming aware of the innate knowledge that you possess, you can begin to tap into this incredible source of wisdom, truth, and strength. The following are some simple steps that will help you to connect with your inner guide:

*1. **Become aware that you have an inner guide in the first place.** We all have a gut instinct or voice inside of us that tells us when something feels good or when things are not right. This is not to be confused with ego or fear. Your inner voice will always have your best interest at heart. Acknowledge that it is there, and try to listen to what it has to say.*

*2. **Start tapping into your true feelings and become aware of any uneasy or opposing emotions that arise from this awareness.** Usually, your first instinct or feeling about a situation or a person will be your true thoughts and feelings. Many people tend to ignore this gut feeling, instead choosing to overthink things until a given situation has been blown out of proportion. Go with your first instinct, and be wary of the root of any conflicting emotions.*

*3. **Meditate.** Meditation allows you to slow down and listen to what your body has to say. By concentrating on your current state of being and drowning out the distractions, you can cultivate a deeper understanding of what your inner guide is trying to tell you.*

*4. **Start asking yourself questions instead of looking for outside help.** For example, you may want to ask yourself, "How do I truly feel about this situation?" or "What can I do in this situation that will result in the best possible outcome for me and for others around me?"*

*5. **Trust what your inner guide is telling you.** Too often, people already know the answer to a question or the solution to a difficult problem, yet they ignore their inner voice and seek external confirmation or advice to deal with it instead. Once you start trusting in yourself, you will most likely find that the decisions you make will result in better outcomes for yourself and for the other people in your life.*

Tapping into your inner guide does not require much work. It is simply a matter of knowing that you have an inner guide, making time to acknowledge this innate wisdom, and trusting what your inner guide has to say.

The purpose here is to make you aware of the importance of constructing a bond with your inner guide as part of your journey toward heart health. After you have learned how to access your inner guide, you can draw on its power at any time.

The voice inside lives within all of us, and we have all likely sensed its presence. It is known as intuition and can serve as an inner guide to direct our decision making and help us attain greater self-knowledge.

Many people are surprised when they connect with their inner guide for the first time. It may be perceived simply as an inner voice, but it can also be experienced as a person, a child, or even an animal. The counsel provided by the inner guide may also be unexpected, perhaps not even what you had hoped to hear. Whether you choose to listen to that counsel is, of course, up to you.

The important thing is making the connection and gaining the ability to become open to the inner person beneath the conscious self. It is a resource that will help you find healing and nurturing for your soul and spirit. If you develop the habit of checking in with that resource every day, you will soon discover that you are able to make better choices about life. Your self-insight will increase and you will start to find greater satisfaction in the outcomes of the choices you have made. When you have established a peaceful and intuitive relationship with the person inside, the inner guide, it will continue to serve as a way to strengthen and nurture your soul and spirit and maintain heart health.

LISTEN TO YOUR DREAMS

THE SUBCONSCIOUS PROMPTING

Anna's younger brother had died unexpectedly and suddenly of cancer. On his birthday a few months later, she had a very powerful dream in which her brother was playing guitar and singing a beautiful song. He kept looking at her and telling her through the lyrics of the song that he was okay. He was happy. Anna woke up from the dream with tears streaming down her face, but feeling a sense of peace that she had not had for a long time.

Mark had a recurring dream of danger and of being attacked by wild animals. Sometimes it would be a tiger stalking from a hidden grove of trees. Other times he would encounter a poisonous snake, waiting to strike. He would feel bites on his arms and they would go numb. He would awaken to a feeling of terror and pressure on his lungs, unable to breathe, gasping for air. Troubled, Mark went for a complete physical, including an EKG. The results indicated that Mark had cardiovascular disease and was at a high risk of heart attack.

Linda kept having disturbing dreams about her granddaughter. In one, the little girl was drowning in a pool of toxic waste. In another, she was falling into a pit of quicksand. The dreams all featured frightening accidents and a fear of loss.

Linda's granddaughter was healthy and there seemed to be no reason for concern. During a family crisis, Linda had an angry confrontation with her daughter and was subsequently not allowed to see her granddaughter for several months. Linda realized that she needed to resolve her fear of losing her granddaughter by building a healthy relationship with her daughter.

Our dreams can be powerful indicators of what is going on inside of us. Many people consider dreams as nothing more than manifestations of tangible emotions we are feeling. They may view dreams as simply the consequence of the brain's organizing the events of each day. Dreams can be all of these things, but they often fall outside the boundaries of rational explanations.

Many people have dreams that have predicted the later development of a medical condition in themselves or their loved ones. Highly creative people have composed great works of art while dreaming. Scientists and mathematicians have worked out complex problems in their dreams.

Given that we sleep an average of eight hours a night and dream for about 25 percent of that time, a significant amount of work is accomplished in those few hours. Dream problem solving is quite common, and research shows that dreams play an important role in consolidating memory, working through trauma, resolving conflict, and regulating mood and emotional health.

Recurring dreams are common, and experts suggest they may point toward significant life issues or things you are concerned about. Nightmares can be a consequence of poor sleep, stress, and anxiety, and they are common in young children between the ages of three and six, when the imagination is at its most active and fears are beginning to develop.

Carl Jung, the famous Swiss psychologist, proposed that dreams reflected psychic activity and, as such, could guide our conscious living. Although you may not believe that dreams are psychic predictors, the reality is that dreams do provide access to our subconscious in a way not usually available to our conscious selves. By providing insight into our subconscious, dreams can guide us not only to things that may be occurring within our physical bodies below our level of conscious awareness, but also to unconscious desires and hopes that we may be suppressing.

Messages sent through dreams are common. Whether you believe these are actual messages or simply a manifestation of some subconscious, inner desire, how you choose to listen to and interpret the notice can have a profound impact on the revitalization of your soul and the health of your heart. To better understand that concept, let's consider the examples we just read.

Anna was processing the loss of her brother. Much of her emotional distress had remained at a subconscious level, and she was unable to mourn openly. On her brother's birthday, these emotions were at the forefront. Her strong desire to believe that her brother was in a better place and free from illness may have led her dreams in that direction. She needed peace and resolution, and because she was able to listen to the dream message, Anna was comforted.

Mark had a stressful job, and he had been experiencing a number of difficult personal issues. He didn't exercise often and was negligent about his diet and self-care. Mark knew he was not taking adequate care of his health and needed some lifestyle changes. Consciously he may have suspected the diagnosis, but he needed the subconscious prompting of his dreams to be the catalyst for action. By listening to the dream message, Mark may have saved his own life.

Linda loved her daughter and granddaughter, but on some level she knew that her relationship with her daughter was shaky. It no doubt contributed to her fear of loss. Her dreams were a reflection of feelings that Linda could not easily accept on the surface—in other words, if she did not find a way to build a healthy relationship with her daughter, she would not be able to sustain a relationship with her granddaughter.

How can we use our dreams to improve our self-knowledge, strengthen the connection with our inner guide, and support better heart health? The quality of our dreams will improve if we have regular sleep patterns and get plenty of good, uninterrupted sleep. External factors play a role. Good and bad smells, for example, are known to cause good or bad dreams. So our sleeping environment should be as restful and comfortable as possible.

Before falling asleep, remind yourself that you want to remember your dreams. Keep a paper and pencil or recording device handy. If you wake up during the night and recall the dream, try to record it right away.

Concentrate on recalling your dream as soon as you wake up. Before moving or getting out of bed, think about the dream and review it in your mind. Do not let any other thoughts intrude. Go through the dream and retell the story, experiencing any accompanying sensations or feelings. As you remember bits and pieces of a scene, relive the dream in reverse, trying to recall what came before. Then record everything you can remember in your dream journal—words, feelings, moods, events, no matter how fragmentary.

With practice, you will become better at recalling what you dreamed. You can then begin to harness the power of your dreams. While there are many resources to help people interpret dreams, in reality, dreams are extremely personal.

There are some commonalities in dreams—being chased, lost, or trapped, falling, public nudity, dying—and some common themes can be identified. Being lost or trapped can represent conflict or facing a difficult choice. Being chased can be some type of physical or emotional threat. These concepts can guide our understanding, but what we dream will relate to our personal situation, and it is not possible to make blanket interpretations.

In understanding your dreams and gaining insight into what the subconscious inner voice is trying to express through them, it is important to have a good sense of your current situation. Consider your job, school, or daily activities, and include the people you interact with. Think about your dreams in the context of those relationships and activities, and include things that may be worrying you: relationships, health problems, life stressors. Consider what message your subconscious may be sending you.

As you draw connections between your dreams and the reality of the situations you are managing in daily life, you will discover that your dreams are a source of valuable insight. Like your inner guide, your dreams can advise you.

Your dreams can make you aware of a potential health issue you may have been ignoring. Your dreams can enlighten you regarding a problem needing resolution. Hidden fears, worries, and vulnerabilities come to light and you can then begin to search for solutions. Your dreams can help you identify suppressed emotions that are leaving you vulnerable to developing heart disease. But are dreams simply a source of insight into the problem, or can they be used in actual problem solving?

LUCID DREAMS

"The sleeper remembers day-life and his own condition, reaches a state of perfect awareness, and is able to direct his attention and to attempt different acts of free volition."

—Frederik Van Eeden, Study of Dreams (1913)

Lucid dreaming is something we experience when we are in a half-awake state and can actually direct the outcome or direction of the dream.

The technique for lucid dreaming is an extension of the process used to recall dreams. Once you have become proficient at remembering the dream, you can learn how to stay in the dream while remaining consciously aware that you are dreaming.

This is not done simply out of a desire to continue a pleasant dream, although that is a very real benefit, but there are heart-health advantages to lucid dreaming. Not only do our dreams often enlighten us as to what might be going on below the surface in our subconscious, but we can use them to direct our subconscious.

To illustrate how it works, take the example of a recurring dream where you are being chased. Perhaps you've already identified the source as a situation where you feel threatened. The person or creature that is chasing you in the dream has been linked to a person or circumstance in real life. But you have not resolved the threat and still feel vulnerable.

In a lucid dream, you can bring that awareness into it. Rather than running, choose to have your dream self turn and face the threat with a weapon or shield in hand. Then you continue the dream to its outcome, whatever it may be. When you are fully awake, you can then explore that outcome and the meaning it might hold for you in finding a resolution to the problem that threatens you.

Some people are naturally quite adept at lucid dreaming. Others learn it through practice. It is another potential tool by which you can connect with your metaphysical heart and spirit.

The messages sent by our subconscious provide a rich source of self-insight. When we don't listen to or communicate with our inner guide, the voices eventually become dormant and stop providing input. Choosing to connect with our inner self will begin the important process of revitalizing and resurrecting the soul and renewing heart health.

THE POWER OF THANK YOU

One of the most powerful expressions in every language around the world is "thank you." We give thanks as a way to show gratitude and appreciation. Saying thank you shows respect and tells others that we value what they have done. It provides encouragement and generates positive emotions for both giver and recipient.

Research has also shown that expressing and receiving thanks has important health benefits. It has been linked with increased energy, enthusiasm, better sleep patterns, and a positive outlook—all things that are important to heart health. Among patients recovering from heart problems, appreciation and thankfulness are predictive of better physical and mental health, along with reduced risk of subsequent cardiovascular events. Loving, appreciative thoughts encourage heart rhythms to maintain a more regular and coherent pattern.

Showing gratitude is important, but to access the spiritual benefits that nurture our soul and spirit, more is involved than simply saying thank you. A daily attitude of gratefulness means being thankful for the basic things in life. If we perceive everything through the lens of gratitude, we can begin to find reasons for thanks in even the most negative or painful occurrence.

The case of Ms. Levine helps illustrate how the experience of death can also be used to celebrate life. Loss of a loved one is sad and tragic, but something valuable can be learned. Philosophers suggest that we need pain and suffering to appreciate the good things in life. Whether this is true or not, we can draw strength and learn from negative events and loss, becoming empowered with gratitude.

Loss can motivate us to find things to be thankful about each day, to pause and appreciate the moment rather than focusing on deadlines to the exclusion of all else. It can remind us to put emphasis on family and friends, to savor each precious moment together. I have a daily practice of identifying five things I am grateful for each morning even before

Research has also shown that expressing and receiving thanks has important health benefits.

I set my feet on the floor. This simple act shifts the entire vibrational mood and sets the tone for the rest of my day.

Showing regular appreciation for the positive aspects of life is linked not only to improved heart health, but also to improved coping skills for dealing with stress and loss, overall psychological well-being, and lowered risk of psychological disorders such as depression.

We can take that a step further and include gratitude for every aspect of life, both positive and negative. Good things in life make us happy and energized. Negative events build resiliency and strength. Positive feedback reinforces self-esteem and guides goal-setting. Negative feedback motivates personal growth and spurs self-improvement.

An attitude of gratefulness energizes heart, soul, and spirit. When we are in the mindset of being appreciative of each single moment, we have the necessary resources to start building the life we truly want.

CREATING THE LIFE YOU WANT

As children, we learn how to love, how to laugh, how to be happy, how to be brave, and how to be creative. As we grow older, we never lose the ability to learn. Even if the toll of daily life seems to have temporarily taken away our laughter and love, these things can be relearned and rebuilt. We can learn to appreciate humor, nature, music, dance, laughter: all the things that energize heart, mind, soul, and spirit and make life enjoyable. It may take some work, but the power to create the lives we want lies within us.

Reflecting on death and dying is one way to learn to create the lives we want. This is not a morbid perspective, but rather a way to look at death as a vehicle for positive change. Our time on Earth is very short, and we have limited opportunities to make our mark. The contributions we make are important, as are the things we leave behind: the people who love us, the memories we have shared, our value as individuals, and the impact we have had on the lives of others. We continue to live forever through the experiences and memories that remain.

In creating the life you want, ask yourself what your legacy will be. Will it be that of a person who chose to live life to the fullest in every possible way? Will you be remembered as someone who knew the value of life and love? Will those memories be filled with a spirit of beauty, gratitude, and love?

A heart that is rested and beating regularly and efficiently, a brain that is functioning to its fullest capacity, a healthy and powerful soul, and an active and engaged spirit—these are the building blocks from which you can create the life you want. Active communication with your inner guide will give you a good sense of who you really are inside. Ponder the wise words of counsel from within. Listen and gain clarity. Choose your next steps to heart health.

Rather than allowing real or imaginary obstacles to get in your way, work for clarity and focus on what really matters to your life. Clean your mind of distractions, slow things down, and spend some time focused on what really matters in your life. Do not stress over what you don't have. Focus on what you do have and find ways to show gratitude for even the smallest blessing. Accept yourself for who you are, and take time each day to love yourself.

If you believe something is impossible, it will be. Rather than believing that happiness and success are impossible, choose to believe that it is impossible not to be happy and successful. That belief will restore your soul. Create joy. Create happiness. Create the life you want to live, and your vibrant heart will follow.

CHAPTER 9

ABCs of a Vibrant Heart

"If you don't like something change it; if you can't change it, change the way you think about it."

—Mary Engelbreit

There is no mysterious secret to creating a vibrant heart and living the life you have always dreamed of. Each of us has the ability to change our lifestyle and the way we think about nutrition, exercise, body chemistry, stress, and peace of mind. The trick is to figure out which areas you need to work on in your life, and then to formulate a plan to reach your chosen goals.

Each of us has the power to make positive changes that will greatly improve our body, mind, and spirit in order to create a life that is long, enjoyable, meaningful, and personally fulfilling.

In the previous chapters, you learned the A to Zs of improving cardiovascular health and avoiding potential diseases and illnesses. Now, let's create action steps that will help you to commit to a better quality of life and to your optimal level of physical, mental, emotional, and spiritual health and well-being.

You can achieve this aim by incorporating what I call the ABC steps of health into your life. ABC stands for Affirmations, Behavior, and

Commitment. These steps are all about taking what you have learned in the previous chapters and applying it to your life to achieve greater health, happiness, and a strong and vibrant heart.

AFFIRMATIONS

To manifest and achieve the life we want to lead and to have the good heart we deserve, positive affirmations are an important and necessary ingredient. Powerful life-changing transformations can be created by expressing positive affirmations and visualizing what we want. This is known as creative visualization.

Like the Universal Law of Attraction, our own subconscious beliefs define our reality. Positive affirmations and positive thinking lead to positive attitudes, which in turn bring love, kindness, gratitude, and other wonderful things into our lives.

Some of the most powerful words to use in an affirmation are "I am," "I can," and "I will." Self-affirmations work like magic because they convey intention and determination. By saying, believing, and delivering these affirmations to ourselves, imagining and creating them, reading them out loud, and writing them down, we are taking ownership of these thoughts and declaring our deepest beliefs and desires to ourselves and to the universe. The more often we state these affirmations, the more empowered we will be.

Affirmations are statements we declare with conviction. They are personal for each individual and most effective when stated with passion. Affirmations should touch us deep down inside. They should excite or even thrill us, and they should make us feel wonderful, refreshed, and revitalized.

Affirmations need to be in the present tense and expressed in a current state of being, and they need to be achievable in our mind and believable in our heart.

> Positive affirmations and positive thinking lead to positive attitudes, which in turn bring love, kindness, gratitude, and other wonderful things into our lives.

Affirmations are often initially met with resistance or negative emotions. It can take some mental effort to reprogram years of negative beliefs and self-doubts. The inner work may seem tremendous, yet in the end it only makes us stronger and more empowered.

The Affirmation of Love

Inner strength and a positive self-image are very important components of overall well-being. The more we respect and love all aspects of ourselves, the better we will treat our bodies, and the happier and healthier we will be.

Some positive affirmations for inner strength and self-image may include statements such as, "I am full of happiness," "I take responsibility for my actions," "I have joy in everything I do," and "I am worth it." These positive statements work to push out anxiety, insecurities, and fear, and they reinforce confidence, accountability, feelings of self-worth, and a positive attitude toward life.

Although we may not realize it, love and relationships contribute a lot to our state of mind, and therefore to our health. Friends, loved ones, and family members can help us improve and maintain mental and emotional health, which reduces harmful stress levels. Sometimes it takes just a few minutes with someone you care about to make you feel lighter and more joyful.

That being said, relationships can be tricky to maintain, and it is all too easy to take the people in our lives for granted. Some positive affirmations to help balance and maintain the important relationships in your life could include, "I respect myself and others," "I am supportive of my friends," "I allow myself to be loved," and "I choose to forgive myself and others."

Affirming Physical Goals

If you have been reading the book up to this point, you know that the body and the mind are not just separate entities working independently of one another. There is a strong connection between the way you think and your overall health, strength, vitality, and willpower. By thinking positive thoughts and encouraging a good outlook on yourself and your abilities, you can achieve almost any fitness goal you put your mind to. In addition, you can even encourage your body to heal faster by thinking positively and raising your vibrational frequency.

For better health, deeper motivation, and increased longevity, you may want to repeat affirmations such as, "I choose to honor my body and allow my body to be my temple," "I enjoy a healthy heart and body," "I am strong enough to reach my goals," and "I exercise self-control over bad habits."

In Western society, the disconnect between the mental and the physical has become a yawning canyon dividing two inextricably intertwined aspects of our health. Yet it is well within our power to reconstruct the bridge between these halves once again. Each affirmation we make toward improving our physical health is a plank in the larger project of that reconstruction and will, ultimately, lead us toward wholeness of health once more.

Affirmations and Your Life's Purpose

In the grand scheme of things, good health, a strong heart, and a positive attitude matter little if you do not understand and celebrate your purpose in life and work toward your own personal success. We are all here for a reason, whether it is to raise a family, create works of art, or save lives. The key to being truly fulfilled and satisfied with your life is to understand your purpose and to strive for success in everything you do.

Sometimes we all need a little kick to remind us of what is important and to motivate us to push past our fears of failure so that each and every one of us can enjoy the life we truly deserve. The following are some of my favorite affirmations to motivate me to live the best possible life I can: "I can create anything I want," "I am uniquely needed in this world," "I choose to release all my fears of failure," and "I am thankful for the smallest things in my past, present, and future."

It is important to choose affirmations for the heart, body, mind, and soul that suit your particular goals or mindset. Pick only one from the area you are working on the most, and use it for a week before moving on to the next. You can tell yourself (either in thought or out loud) the affirmation whenever you think of it, say it to yourself when you wake up or every hour, write it down on small pieces of paper that you post on your bathroom mirror and around your living space, and write about the affirmation before going to sleep each night.

After the first week, pick another affirmation from that same section or alternate with affirmations from the four areas of life you want to strengthen. Over time, your mind will incorporate these new ways of thinking. Soon your heart, mind, and soul will respond with greater feelings of health, pride, joy, self-worth, and self-confidence.

Daily affirmations will raise your energetic vibration and will become incorporated into your very essence and being. You can receive my free e-book *101 Positive Affirmations to Revitalize-U* by visiting www.drcynthia.com/affirmations.

BEHAVIOR

One of the most important steps in the journey toward a healthier and happier life and a vibrant heart is the way you choose to behave with respect to your body, mind, and soul. When it comes down to it, you are the only one who is responsible for the way you live your life. You can choose to honor your body and make healthy decisions that will benefit your overall well-being, or you can choose to continue taking part in behavior that you know is harmful to your health.

Making behavioral changes can be challenging, particularly in the beginning. Old habits are hard to break, and sometimes just getting started is the most difficult part.

Setting Goals

The first step in changing any type of behavior is to think about your goals, both short-term and long-term. Think about what type of life you truly want to live, the level of health and fitness you would like to have, and the person you want to be.

An important guideline in setting your goals is to not limit your true potential by selling yourself short. Far too many people do not achieve their goals because they do not think them achievable or because they do not already know how to achieve them. The key to remember is this: assuring a successful outcome is not your responsibility. You are responsible only for setting your goals and taking appropriate action steps toward achieving those goals.

Write your goals down and post them in a place where you can see them every day. Then try to formulate a plan for how you are going to achieve those goals. Organize your time so that you can fit in exercise, time to prepare healthy meals, and quality time for yourself. Try to predict any obstacles that you may come across in achieving your goals and how you will tackle those obstacles.

Be realistic when you are forming your plan. For example, it may be a nice idea to

> Assuring a successful outcome is not your responsibility. You are responsible only for setting your goals and taking appropriate action steps toward achieving those goals.

lose forty pounds in one month, but that simply is not going to happen. The more honest you are with yourself, and the better prepared you are, the more likely you will be to succeed.

Practice Patience

Forming and practicing new behaviors is rarely easy, particularly if you have been working within the constraints of old habits for years. Regardless of whether you are approaching healthy eating habits, physical exercise, or mental clarity, there will more than likely be times when it feels as though you are taking two steps forward and one step back. At times like these, patience becomes the deciding factor between those who are able to follow through with the creation of a vibrant heart and those who aren't.

For many of us, it is far easier to practice patience with others than it is to bestow it on ourselves. Yet forgiving our own weaknesses is the key that will allow us to overcome those weaknesses at the end of the day. Although the rewards of a vibrant heart are rich and manifold, we must accept from the beginning that the path to ultimate health may not be an easy one to travel.

For instance, although you know intellectually that going through a detox program will benefit you in the end, you may find that you go through emotional withdrawals or regressions when you begin the process. A friend of mine knew a man who, when he started going through detox, smelled like tobacco for a month even though he had stopped smoking ten years earlier. When the aches, pains, or other unpleasant side effects begin to appear, and when you are feeling at your worst, you may be tempted to give up on the process altogether.

These are the moments when practicing self-patience will mean the difference between success and failure. Be kind to yourself. Remind yourself that the path you have chosen is not easy, and that it is normal to experience moments of discouragement. Then refocus your awareness on your goals, pick yourself up, and put your best foot forward once again.

Start Small

The best thing to do when you are first beginning to establish new behaviors is to start small. Take manageable steps that are achievable, and then gradually introduce additional changes after you have mastered each previous task.

For example, if your goal is to exercise more, start with short, mild workout sessions a few days a week. Remember that Rome was not built in a day. It takes time to achieve your goals, so be patient with and kind to yourself, and realize that even the smallest steps can make a huge difference in transforming your quality of life.

To achieve optimum health and a strong heart, it may be necessary to work on many areas of your life. In today's fast-paced society, the majority of people around the world could benefit from a healthier diet, more exercise, and less stress. However, it is important not to attempt to change too many things in your life all at once. Start by introducing one change at a time, and concentrate on putting your energy and time into that one change.

I want to introduce the concept of the 6:1 method, taught to me by my mentor, Mary Morrissey. To advance your goal and your vision, make a concrete decision to devote a period of time toward advancing that goal daily (it could be ten minutes or two hours, but consistency is the key).

Make a list of six action steps that will advance that goal, and prioritize them in rank of importance. Then each day, spend the allotted time you have dedicated toward achieving the first item on your list, and only move on to item two on the list after you have achieved item one. The items on the list should make up a "to do" list of easily achievable action steps, not a "to be" list, which consists of more long-term commitments.

Take note of what this simple practice of taking action does toward advancing your goal. Take note of the achievement and of the accomplishments. Take note of the positive state of your being. Do not pay attention to any difficulties you encounter along the way. Do not give the slightest energy to the negative state, to the old habits, or to the previous conditions. Instead, reward yourself for your accomplishments, and recognize any positive results in your fitness level, appearance, or overall feeling of well-being.

Once you have successfully introduced a new, positive behavior into your day-to-day routine, or vanquished a bad habit, then you can move on to the next positive change in your life. The key is always forward movement, one step at a time.

Find Support

Although your health rests largely upon your own shoulders, the people around you can offer a great deal of support as you work toward building your optimal lifestyle. Do not be afraid to ask for help from friends, family members, or even support groups in your community or online. The people who truly love you will be excited that you are making positive changes in your life, and they will most likely be extremely supportive of the efforts you make to improve your quality of life.

In addition, other people who are also trying to transform their lives can share their stories with you, give you much-needed advice, or act as a sounding board for any difficulties you may be having. Remember that you are not alone in your efforts, and that there are many other people out there who are also hoping for you to succeed in creating a healthy and happy life.

Friends, family, and support groups are great for those of us who need a little boost in self-confidence or someone to lean on. However, some of us can also benefit greatly from professional help.

If you suffer from cardiovascular disease, metabolic syndrome, diabetes, hypertension, or another life-threatening illness, I highly recommend that you get medical advice from a health-care professional before embarking on a self-improvement quest. A physician can give you valuable information about how to eat properly, exercise safely, and decrease stress levels in ways that are appropriate for your particular condition.

In addition, nutritionists, personal trainers, and meditation instructors are just a few examples of people who can help you get on the right track toward optimum health and well-being. These experts can give you the basics of positive lifestyle practices while teaching you the proper methods of doing things so that you can build on those methods yourself in the future. Setting a solid foundation for your health and vitality just makes good sense.

COMMITMENT

If you are like 99 percent of people out there, then there are times in your life you can remember when you set goals and, for whatever reason, gave up on those goals.

Perhaps you wanted to master a musical instrument, quit your job and follow your dreams, stop smoking, or lose a significant amount of weight. Maybe you were initially excited and motivated about the desired outcome. Perhaps you even set a plan in place and made a blueprint for how to succeed. In the beginning you made a real effort to succeed, but as time went on you gradually contributed less and less effort to achieving that goal, and finally you stopped trying altogether.

There are many reasons why people choose not to commit to their goals. Distractions, obstacles, and fear of failure are all contributing factors when it comes to giving up on plans. To truly achieve better health and a greater sense of overall well-being, it is crucial that you commit to your goals.

Defining True Commitment

Mary tells a story of her recent decision to commit to improving her health by starting a walking program. While it was difficult to incorporate this new practice into her busy schedule of coaching, lectures, and speaking engagements, Mary thought she was doing quite well given the circumstances. Several weeks into her new activity, a friend called and inquired about her success. Mary informed her friend with pride that she was walking four days a week. Her friend proceeded to ask her how committed she was to achieving her goal of improved health. Mary responded 70 percent, but then it dawned on her that a true "commitment" would be all or nothing.

There was no such thing as a 50 percent or 70 percent commitment. Mary did not commit to faithfulness in her marriage 70 percent of the time. Activities such as brushing her teeth or taking daily showers were not negotiable habits. As such, she realized that to achieve her goal and attain her vision, she had to make a 100 percent commitment to walking.

While it makes perfect sense to break your goals down into small, step-by-step achievements, commitment does not work the same way. Your commitment to your health is the foundation upon which your goals—small and large alike—will find support and security. Just as stars cannot exist without a dark sky behind them, a vibrant heart cannot be achieved unless your commitment to yourself is absolute.

Overcoming Obstacles

When you are in the midst of transforming your behavior to benefit your body, mind, and spirit, it can be easy to lose sight of the bigger picture. Obstacles may arise that make it difficult to progress and easy to simply throw in the towel. This is when it is important to remember why you are making these changes in the first place.

One of the best things you can do for yourself is to write down your goals and your reasons for wanting to achieve these goals. Perhaps you have children and you want to be around long enough to watch them grow and thrive. Maybe you have already had a cardiac episode, and you realize that you need to make some serious life changes if you want to avoid more health problems. Or perhaps you simply want to lose a few pounds so that you look and feel better. Whatever your motivation, it helps to remind yourself of what you truly want and why so that you stay on track and committed.

There are times when staying committed to your health and to yourself may seem to become entangled in the complications of day-to-day life. For example, my personal commitment to improve my nutrition sometimes found itself at odds with the wider expectation that I would eat traditional cultural foods during family events and celebrations. Especially in the beginning, it was difficult to keep myself on track because of the feeling I had that I was saying "no" not just to friends and family, but to my entire culture.

The pressures we receive from others and from society as a whole to conform to certain expectations can exert a powerful effect on us, particularly in social settings. At moments like these, remember that your personal responsibility is first and foremost to yourself. In due time, those who insist that you should be acting otherwise will see for themselves that the transformation you are bringing about in yourself is ultimately not just for your own benefit, but also for the benefit of everyone around you.

What many people do not know or choose to ignore about obstacles is the fact that the way you experience life is highly dependent on how you perceive the world around you. This means that if you choose to believe that you are too busy to exercise, to eat healthy, nutritious foods, or to de-stress, then you ultimately will be. Likewise, if you choose to believe that something is just too difficult or impossible, then it will become the case.

However, if you make the conscious decision to improve your lifestyle, to not let outside influences or self-destructive thought patterns stop you from reaching your goals, and to be proactive and positive in everything you do, you will find that you can achieve anything you set your mind to. A good way to stay focused and committed is to remind yourself each morning that you have the power to choose how you will let life's obstacles affect you. Remember that it is you who makes your life what it is, and that you also have the power to decide how you want to live your life.

My Renewed Commitment:
Overcoming the Obstacles to a Healthy Diet

I have faced my share of obstacles in effecting positive change in myself and in my family. Food is one example. Since watching the documentary *Forks Over Knives*, I had been contemplating the idea of adopting a plant-based diet. I had just completed my trial of the Ideal Protein protocol and was beginning to transition back to a normal diet. I had learned enough about my physical and spiritual self to appreciate the delicate balance between my choice of foods and my general sense of health. My body felt light and unencumbered after undergoing the detoxification process.

Yet while all the knowledge and science was there, and my motivation was strong, the actual day-to-day process of planning and preparing meals, along with the challenge of retraining my children's palates after years of not-so-great eating, felt like an obstacle that was just too high for me to master. Consequently, for a while I succumbed to the comfort and ease of what was familiar.

But where the will is strong, a way will be found. For me, that way was the Farms 2 Forks immersion weekend. The three days I spent there, listening to fascinating in-depth lectures, watching educational demonstrations, and eating healthy food, changed everything for me. The retreat gave me the practical tools I needed to succeed—such as cooking demonstrations on fifteen-minute plant-strong and nutritionally balanced meals, and an ongoing support structure provided by Rip Esselstyn and his team— and I duly noted them all down.

Rip himself, a former firefighter-turned-dragon-slayer battling the evils of the standard American diet and the obesity epidemic, was inspiring. I finally realized that commitment was no longer beyond my reach. By taking action to attend the conference, I had shifted my goal back into my circle of control, and everything I needed to achieve it had been there waiting for me.

Make Your Commitment Public

Another way to stay committed to your goals is to go public with them. By declaring to the universe your intention, you increase your chances of success, because the universe becomes energetically aligned with that vision.

In addition, by telling other people what you hope to achieve, you create a network of support and accountability. This way other people can keep you motivated and committed to your efforts. You will be less likely to give up on your goals if you know that other people are keeping an eye on you and rooting for you to succeed.

Involving other people in your life transformation does not mean that you have to ask people to babysit you or monitor your progress. It may be as simple as joining a group fitness class, where other people will encourage you to challenge yourself and notice if you miss a large number of classes.

You may want to create a buddy system with someone who has similar goals to you, or ask your spouse or family members to call you out if you slip back into old habits. No matter how many people you involve, you will be less likely to give up on your goals if you know others are watching you and supporting your efforts.

The One-Degree Shift

Whenever I talk to patients about making changes to their lifestyles—whether with regard to their diets, exercise habits, or anything else—they think they need to make drastic changes right off the bat. Because the magnitude of the commitment before them seems overwhelming, they are unable to bring themselves to take the first step: their intimidation results in no movement at all, and their situations cannot improve.

In such cases, I explain to my patients that the change I am encouraging them to make does not need to happen drastically. All I am asking of them is a one-degree shift in their mindset, in their commitment, and in their actions. If they can commit to that one-degree shift on a daily basis, then thirty or sixty days later the trajectory of their lives and their health will have seen a dramatic shift without a dramatic upheaval in their daily routines.

So what, then, constitutes a one-degree shift? The wonderful thing about this process is that its steps can often be deceptively simple, such as committing to trying one new vegetable a week, or taking a ten-minute walk. The key to making the one-degree shift work is constant forward movement, or at the very least maintaining the commitment level that you are at.

There must be no backsliding. If you commit to walking ten minutes daily, you must be consistent about that commitment. Then, when you are ready, add another ten minutes to your routine, but remember: now you need to consistently walk twenty minutes daily. You cannot take a day off and revert to ten minutes again, as that will undermine the whole undertaking.

The problem that most patients face is that they start out trying to commit to more change than is realistically sustainable. Then, when they are inevitably forced to stop, they become discouraged because they did not give themselves the full opportunity to see results. However, if you take life's large challenges in small steps, shifting just one degree at a time, success will bloom and flourish right beneath your feet.

Change

The definition of change is to replace with another or shift from one to another. It is very empowering to recognize that everything that exists in nature, including our very essence, is fluid and in constant flux. The notion that our current reality is not fixed and that the potential for change exists within the very fabric of our DNA should inspire us to recognize and seize the opportunity. Commitment to self-recognition and self-development is the start of that change.

If you truly want to change, your brain knows exactly what needs to take place. Change begins with liberation of the mind to connect with the creative consciousness, trust in the inner guide, and not let judgment and self-doubt stand in the way.

True change is attainable to all. For me, it starts with following the teaching of the Buddha's Noble Eightfold Path to enlightenment. Four elements are the essence or core necessary to accomplish any change you would like in life: right mindfulness, right thought, right speech, and right action.

What we think, what we say, and what we do, along with being acutely aware of our present moment, will determine our success or failure with the change that we commit to.

To further your understanding, I would encourage you to view the documentary *Change: The LifeParticle Effect* and read its companion book, *Change: Realizing Your Greatest Potential*, both created by Ilchi Lee. The main messages of the film and the book are that everything exists as potential, reality is changeable, and that we have the power to change. True understanding of this simple perspective will change how you view the world and your circumstances and how you choose to relate to external events. This film and book will change how you navigate through your life.

Overcoming the Fear of Failure

One of the main reasons that people give up on their dreams is a fear of failure. It can be a daunting task to make significant life changes, regardless of how positive those changes can be. However, as the saying goes, the only thing standing in the way of your success is you. It is all too easy to look at one challenge or one mistake and convince yourself that you cannot do something. Negative thinking can drastically reduce your chances of achieving the life that you truly deserve.

Try to be kind to yourself and think positively. This is where affirmations can really help. Start your day by reminding yourself of your goal, how strong and capable you are, and how committed you are to the end result. If you think positively and keep an open mind, there is nothing you cannot achieve.

Just as it is important to think positively and be kind to yourself, it is also important not to beat yourself up if you make a mistake or get off track. Nobody gets everything right all the time, and mistakes are a normal part of human nature. If you have a day where you slip up and eat food that you know is unhealthy, skip an exercise session, or allow stress to overwhelm you, it is not the end of the world. Simply recognize what caused you to stray from your path, create a method for how to deal with that obstacle if and when it arises in the future, and get on up and try again.

True commitment means sticking to your lifestyle plan, regardless of setbacks. In my opinion, mistakes are a necessary part of life, and they only make us stronger and wiser in the long run. Think of your mistakes as learning experiences, and use the knowledge you gain from them to make yourself even stronger and more successful.

By practicing the ABCs of a vibrant heart—Affirmations, Behavior, and Commitment—you will create the firm foundation you need to push your health beyond the limits of crisis response. You will lift it up to new levels of recovery, strength, and personal fulfillment. And where the heart goes, the rest of life must follow.

CHAPTER 10

BEYOND A VIBRANT HEART

"I slept and dreamt that life was joy. I awoke and saw that life was service. I acted and behold, service was joy."

—Rabindranath Tagore

Ultimately, having a fulfilling life extends further than the simple possession of good health. It rises to heights far beyond that, and it does so with the ongoing cultivation of a vibrant heart. This is because a vibrant heart does not just live. A vibrant heart thrives.

A staggering number of people in our society live in a state of depression and negativity. We see the effects of them every day on both a small scale and a larger one, like dominoes: from the driver cutting us off at our exit on the freeway to the tragic school shootings that are becoming a growing epidemic in our nation. One unhappy person will inspire a similar attitude in those who cross his or her path and, like a contagious flu, the unhappiness spreads.

Negativity, like its positive counterpart, is a choice. I believe that it is in our power as individuals to reverse this domino effect for the better. When that driver cuts you off at your exit, you can make the decision to give in to road rage and push the same frustration on to the next driver, or you can choose a path of kindness and forgiveness and allow that next driver a spot in your lane when the turn you both need is coming up. You can become bitter and vengeful at the news of horrific shootings, or you can roll up your sleeves and contribute to the cause to end gun violence. One of those

> Together, through simple acts of kindness and statements of gratitude and appreciation, we have the power to collectively raise the bar of humanity.

choices fuels the fire that sparked the violence in the first place. The other works toward quelling it for the safety of future generations.

Together, through simple acts of kindness and statements of gratitude and appreciation, we have the power to collectively raise the bar of humanity. Our vibrant hearts can be the catalysts for a new ripple effect: one that promotes love and peace in the world rather than the current trends of anger and mistrustfulness.

My small gesture of kindness to that other driver on the road may in turn inspire him or her to pass it along to someone else. The empowering information I share with one of my patients may end up being something that she then carries on to share with her employees. This is the trail of dominoes that inspires positive change in the world. We as a community can rise to face the challenges of our day, simply by fostering a more conscious level of awareness in the way we live our lives.

Yet while the reach of our positive influence may be limitless, we must never forget to nurture the source of it all: ourselves.

THE INFINITE POTENTIAL OF YOUR PERSONAL VIBRANT HEART

A movement is only as strong as the individuals who fill its ranks. Far too often, we know the people around us—spouses, children, friends, and parents—like the back of our hand, yet the backs of our own hands remain unknown to us. Before anything can happen on a larger scale, it must happen on an individual one.

Most people in our culture look toward medicine or surgery as the answer to their health problems. But these things can only help us cope with the symptoms of the problems we face. The answer to true health really lies in loving yourself, in loving others, and in cultivating your vibrant heart so that you are able to put yourself in a place of service to others without taxing your own mental and physical health. When you achieve this balance, the fundamental physiology of your body changes. Anxiety, inflammation, wayward hormones, and any number of other bad symptoms clear away or hibernate.

Each of us must find this balance with the world so that we can develop a deeper appreciation of who we are. Each of us must discover the potency of that appreciation. Only then will we be able to watch the magic of true healing unfold within ourselves.

One story that I like to tell is that of Lester Levenson, founder of the Sedona Method of meditation. At the age of forty-two, Lester suffered his second massive heart attack, and that in combination with myriad other health issues left his doctors at a loss. They told him that he had six months to live and sent him home to die.

At first, Lester was enraged by this. But then he began to think. What was it, he asked himself, that made him truly happy in life? By the world's standards, he was the epitome of success: a physicist and a successful entrepreneur with a penthouse on New York's Central Park South. Yet his flourishing career did not make him happy. Then he thought that perhaps it was the love of other people that made him happy, but that was not true either: people did love him, but he was still unhappy.

Finally, the realization came to him that it was not the things of the world that gave him happiness. Rather, it was his personal contribution to the world, born of his own internal love, that filled him with the greatest sense of fulfillment.

As soon as he acknowledged this, everything changed for Lester. He released his anger and his negativity, and he forgave the doctors and everyone else who he felt had wronged him. He moved to Sedona, where he started a rehabilitation center for those whose situations resembled his own.

The results of this shift speak for themselves. Instead of six months, Lester Levenson lived another forty years after his supposedly terminal diagnosis. Most importantly, he lived those years in true happiness and fulfillment, pursuing his life's purpose and fueled by a strong sense of inner appreciation and love.

Not everyone has a story this dramatic to tell. Nevertheless, like Lester, the creation of your vibrant heart is a journey that will be unique to you. As you navigate through life, you may discover that the specific tools and techniques that serve you best are combinations or variations of the raw ideas you've read here. Use these ideas as catalysts to push yourself to explore and experiment, but do not box yourself in by feeling that you must follow every rule and instruction to the letter.

Learning to internalize the methods that have been laid out in these pages is the essence of achieving a vibrant heart. To witness their evolution in a way that is original and meaningful to you is to know that you are following your true life purpose, and that you are constructing an individual path to health and happiness that is meant to be traveled by you alone.

The ways that different people tailor and combine the lessons of creating a vibrant heart are endlessly diverse. For instance, perhaps one facet of your personal goal is to become more physically fit, yet you are not keen on traditional methods of exercise. On the other hand, you feel mentally uplifted when you create opportunities for social interaction in your life. In that case, you might consider signing up for a dance class, thereby merging your emotional health with an activity that will also push you toward achieving your goal of physical fitness.

Or perhaps you're hoping to improve your diet, but you derive a lot of joy from throwing fun parties for your friends on Saturday nights. In that case, you could think about setting an organic food theme for those parties in order to satisfy both the physical and the spiritual requirements of your intentions at once.

These combinations do not need to be complex. They only need to be effective. A friend of mine knows a woman who meditates when she goes swimming in the morning. The possibilities go on and on.

MIND-BODY AXIS

H.E.A.R.T.

The mnemonic **HEART** *will remind you of all that is necessary to create the vision, set the course, and manifest the health you have always desired for yourself.*

H *stands for heart. What would you love? What is the health you desire?*

E *stands for emotions. Emotions are the gateway to your subconscious and will be your inner guide to determine if your stated purpose or goal is truly aligned with your inner self.*

A *stands for action. According to Wallace Wattles in* The Science of Getting Rich, *"By thought, the thing you want is brought to you, by action, you receive it. Whatever your action is to be, it is evident that you must act now. You cannot act in the past and it is essential to the clearness of your mental vision that you dismiss the past from your mind, and you cannot act in the future, as the future is not here yet . . . Act now." Do all that you can do today.*

R *stands for reflected reality. Our reality is a perfect reflection of our current predominant thinking pattern. So if you are not content with your current reality, change your dominant thinking pattern.*

T *stands for thanks. Deep and profound gratitude allows for constant positive vibrational energy. Start each day by thinking about five things you are thankful for in your life. Remind yourself of these things throughout the day. You will find that your life seems a lot more cheerful when you remind yourself of the good in it.*

I myself have gone through many stages in the personal evolution of my unique vibrant heart. Starting with the step of tracing my mental growth all the way back to my mother's roots as a healer in Myanmar, I have pursued my personal journey through times of struggle and hardship, adapted as I have deemed necessary, and blossomed from my experiences as a result.

My own personal tapestry of balance fills me with strength and with the daily blessing of deep fulfillment. You, too, have the power to define and achieve your aspirations by adapting the simple actions of everyday life into the reality that you have been envisioning for yourself.

Evolution through the personal awareness of our physical, mental, and spiritual health is essential as we continue to propel ourselves down the path of expanding wellness. As you progress toward striking a balance of healthy habits that is unique to you, pay attention to the small blessings and rewards that begin to sprout from your efforts. Whether those translate into little pockets of excess fat disappearing from your frame, or into unexpected moments of tranquility in the midst of a bustling day, all the signs you need to affirm the rightness of each new step of your personal journey will be there for you, day by passing day.

EXPANDING POSSIBILITIES

The effects of a strong physical, mental, and spiritual heart do not stop where health ends and the rest of existence begins. Your vibrant heart is the first step toward creating your vibrant life. Your vibrant life is the catalyst that will create a vibrant world not only for yourself, but also for those you know and care about.

Many of you reading these pages may be recovering from a life-threatening situation. Yet the knowledge you have just received is not limited to suggestions for averting crises. Far from it. It is the fabric we must all use moving forward to weave a foundation that will forgo the need for crises altogether.

The more you continue to use the tools and opportunities available to you by changing your habits and making a positive difference in your life, the more those good choices will begin to compound themselves. As you grow stronger as an individual, you will notice that you are beginning to affect the people around you in positive ways as well, including your children, your friends, your partner, and your work colleagues. You will experience more peace and joy on an internal level, and that joy will radiate out into the world around you, much as it did for me.

 Cultivating a vibrant heart is a rewarding and an ongoing process. Connecting with those on similar journeys is a wonderful way to keep your motivation strong and your horizons expanding. You will find the resources you need to continue your journey on my website (www.drcynthia.com), where we provide upcoming news, events, and workshops supporting your vibrant heart.

 My personal joy and passion in my line of work come from hearing and sharing the stories of my patients. I would love to hear from you and help you on your personal journey toward a vibrant heart. Share your stories on our forum at www.yourvibrantheart.com.

Celebrate the magnificence of your exquisite heart and pay tribute to the miracle of creation of this splendid organ and all that it represents. The heart is more than just a physical organ. It is the essence of life, providing us with bottomless enrichment and giving meaning, emotion, and spirit to our existence.

To maintain heart health is to engage in a rich and vibrant life filled with love, laughter, awareness, personal responsibility, and enlightenment.

Through these simple acts, each of us holds the power not only to restore our physical and emotional health, but also to make our lives blossom in ways that border the very edges of our imaginations and beyond. Each of us holds the power not just to live, but also to thrive. Each of us holds the incredible power of our own vibrant heart!

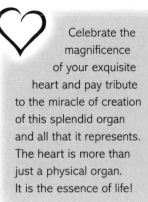

Celebrate the magnificence of your exquisite heart and pay tribute to the miracle of creation of this splendid organ and all that it represents. The heart is more than just a physical organ. It is the essence of life!

About Dr. Cynthia Thaik

Dr. Cynthia Thaik is a Harvard-trained cardiologist specializing in women's health, cardiovascular health, and congestive heart failure. She is the founder of Revitalize-U: A New Body Image, a wellness center focused on health, nutrition, weight loss, and detoxification.

She has served as the co-director of the Women's Cardiac Risk Screening Program at Providence Saint Joseph Medical Center and as the assistant clinical professor of medicine at the University of California, Los Angeles School of Medicine. Among her recognitions are the National Institute of Health's National Research Service Award, the American College of Cardiology's Cardiovascular Research Award, and the Raymond Kalil Memorial Cardiovascular Research Award.

A practicing Buddhist, Dr. Thaik believes in being centered and present in each moment. She teaches that each individual has the amazing potential to heal ailments through mindfulness. On a mission to shift the medical paradigm from crisis management to maintaining wellness, Dr. Thaik has helped thousands of patients take purposeful action to transform their health through the way they think, feel, and act. A strong believer in personal responsibility, Dr. Cynthia doesn't just prescribe these practices to her patients; she incorporates them into her daily family life, as well. She lives in the Los Angeles area with her husband and her three children.

Selected Recommended Readings and Resources

Allen, James. 2013. *As a Man Thinketh*. Tribeca Books.

Lipton, Bruce H., Ph.D. 2008. *The Biology of Belief: Unleashing the Power of Consciousness, Matter, & Miracles*. Hay House.

Robbins, John. 1998. *Diet for a New America: How Your Food Choices Affect Your Health, Happiness and the Future of Life on Earth*. HJ Kramer.

Ornish, Dean, M.D. 1995. *Dr. Dean Ornish's Program for Reversing Heart Disease: The Only System Scientifically Proven to Reverse Heart Disease Without Drugs or Surgery*. Ivy Books.

Barnard, Neal, M.D. 2008. *Dr. Neal Barnard's Program for Reversing Diabetes: The Scientifically Proven System for Reversing Diabetes without Drugs*. Rodale Books.

Esselstyn, Rip. 2009. *The Engine 2 Diet: The Texas Firefighter's 28-Day Save-Your-Life Plan that Lowers Cholesterol and Burns Away the Pounds*. Grand Central Life & Style.

Fuhrman, Joel, M.D. 2008. *Eat for Health: Lose Weight, Keep It Off, Look Younger, Live Longer*. Gift of Health Press.

Ornish, Dean, M.D. 2000. *Eat More, Weigh Less: Dr. Dean Ornish's Life Choice Program for Losing Weight Safely While Eating Abundantly*. William Morrow.

Fuhrman, Joel, M.D. 2011. *Eat to Live: The Revolutionary Formula for Fast and Sustained Weight Loss*. Little, Brown and Company. Revised edition.

Fuhrman, Joel, M.D. 2012 *The End of Diabetes*. Harper Collins Publishers.

Kabat-Zinn, Jon, Ph.D. 1990. *Full Catastrophe Living: Using the Wisdom of Your Body and Mind to Face Stress, Pain, and Illness*. Delta.

Sinatra, Stephen T. 1999. *Heartbreak and Heart Disease: A Mind/Body Prescription for Healing the Heart.* I B S Books Stocked. Second edition.

Siegel, Bernie, M.D. 1998. *Love, Medicine and Miracles: Lessons Learned about Self-Healing from a Surgeon's Experience with Exceptional Patients.* William Morrow.

Haanel, Charles. 2013. *The Master Key System.* SoHo Books.

McDougall, John A. 1998. *The McDougall Program for a Healthy Heart: A Life-Saving Approach to Preventing and Treating Heart Disease.* Plume.

Kabat-Zinn, Jon, Ph.D. 2011. *Mindfulness for Beginners: Reclaiming the Present Moment—and Your Life.* Sounds True. Har/Com edition.

Tolle, Eckhart. 2004. *The Power of Now: A Guide to Spiritual Enlightenment.* New World Library.

Borysenko, Joan, Ph.D., and Miroslav Borysenko, Ph.D. 1994. *The Power of the Mind to Heal.* Hay House, Inc.

Esselstyn, Jr., Caldwell B., M.D. 2008. *Prevent and Reverse Heart Disease: The Revolutionary, Scientifically Proven, Nutrition-Based Cure.* Avery Trade.

Sears, William, M.D. 2010. *Prime-Time Health: A Scientifically Proven Plan for Feeling Young and Living Longer.* Little, Brown and Company.

Smith, Jeffrey M. 2003. *Seeds of Deception: Exposing Industry and Government Lies About the Safety of the Genetically Engineered Foods You're Eating.* Yes Books. Third edition.

Engdahl, William F. 2007. *Seeds of Destruction: The Hidden Agenda of Genetic Manipulation.* Global Research.

Hyman, Mark. 2009. *The UltraMind Solution.* Scribner.

Pritchett, Price. 2007. *You 2: A High Velocity Formula for Multiplying Your Personal Effectiveness in Quantum Leaps.* Pritchett & Associates.

Organizations/Websites

American College of Cardiology: www.acc.org

American Diabetes Association: www.diabetes.org

American Heart Association: www.heart.org

American Heart Association Nutrition Center:
www.heart.org/HEARTORG/GettingHealthy/NutritionCenter/
Nutrition-Center_UCM_001188_SubHomePage.jsp

American Medical Association: www.ama-assn.org

Centers for Disease Control and Prevention: www.cdc.gov

Harvard Health Publications: www.health.harvard.edu

Heart and Stroke Foundation: www.heartandstroke.com

Mayo Clinic | Healthy Lifestyle:
www.mayoclinic.com/health/HealthyLivingIndex/HealthyLivingIndex

National Center for Health Statistics: www.cdc.gov/nchs

National Diabetes Education Program: www.ndep.nih.gov

National Heart, Lung, and Blood Institute: www.nhlbi.nih.gov

National Institutes of Health: www.nih.gov

Nutrition Security Institute: www.nutritionsecurity.org

Physicians Committee for Responsible Medicine: www.pcrm.org

ScienceDaily: www.sciencedaily.com

The Tapping Solution: www.thetappingsolution.com

The World's Healthiest Foods: www.whfoods.org

Movies

Dirt! The Movie. Directed by Bill Benenson. 2009.

Fat, Sick & Nearly Dead. Directed by Joe Cross. 2011.

Food Fight. Directed by Christopher Taylor. 2008.

Food, Inc. Directed by Robert Kenner. 2009.

Food Matters. Directed by James Colquhoun. 2008.

Forks Over Knives. Directed by Lee Fulkerson. 2011.

The Future of Food. Directed by Deborah Koons. 2004.

Genetic Roulette: The Gamble of Our Lives. Directed by Jeffrey M. Smith. 2012.

Change: The LifeParticle Effect. Directed by Edwin Kim, E.J. 2013.

Hungry for Change. Directed by James Colquhoun. 2012.

Killer at Large: Why Obesity Is America's Greatest Threat. Directed by Steven Greenstreet. 2008.

King Corn. Directed by Aaron Woolf. 2007.

The Tapping Solution. Directed by Nick Ortner. 2009.

What's on Your Plate? Directed by Catherine Gund. 2009.

You Can Heal Your Life. Directed by Michael A. Goorjian. 2009.

Bibliography

Chapter 1

Jiang, W., and J. R. Davidson. 2005. "Antidepressant therapy in patients with ischemic heart disease." *American Heart Journal* 150(5) (November): 871–81.

Frasure-Smith, N., F. Lespérance, and M. Talajic. 1993. "Depression following myocardial infarction: Impact on 6-month survival." *JAMA* 270(15) (October 20): 1819–25.

Ruo, B., J. S. Rumsfeld, M. A. Hlatky, H. Liu, W. S. Browner, and M. A. Whooley. 2003. "Depressive symptoms and health-related quality of life: The Heart and Soul study." *JAMA* 290(2) (July 9): 215–21.

Lichtman, J. H., J. T. Bigger, J. A. Blumenthal, N. Frasure-Smith, P. G. Kaufmann, F. Lespérance, et al. 2008. "Depression and coronary heart disease: Recommendations for screening, referral and treatment." A science advisory from the American Heart Association Prevention Committee of the Council on Cardiovascular Nursing, Council on Clinical Cardiology, Council on Epidemiology and Prevention, and Interdisciplinary Council on Quality of Care and Outcomes Research: endorsed by the American Psychiatric Association. *Circulation* 118(17) (October 21): 1768–75.

Berkman, L. F., J. Blumenthal, M. Burg, R. M. Carney, D. Catellier, M. J. Cowan, S. M. Czajkowski, et al. 2003. "Effects of treating depression and low perceived social support on clinical events after myocardial infarction: The Enhancing Recovery in Coronary Heart Disease patients (ENRICHD) randomized trial." *JAMA* 289(23): 3106–16.

Dinan, Timothy G. 2009. "Inflammatory markers in depression." Department of Psychiatry and Alimentary Pharmabiotic Centre, University College Cork, Cork, Ireland. *Curr Opin Psychiatry* 22: 32–6.

Regnante, Richard A., Ryan W. Zuzek, Syed R. Latif, Russell A. Linsky, Hanna N. Ahmed, and Immad Sadiq. 2009. "Clinical characteristics and four-year outcomes of patients in the Rhode Island Takotsubo Cardio-myopathy Registry." *American Journal of Cardiology*. April.

Moorman, Antoon F., and Vincent M. Christoffels. 2003. "Cardiac Chamber Formation: Development, Genes, and Evolution." *Physiol Rev.* 83: 1223–1267.

Chapter 2

Kochanek, K. D., J. Xu, S. L. Murphy, A. M. Miniño, and H. C. Kung. 2011. "Deaths: Final data for 2009." National Vital Statistics System. *National Vital Statistics Reports* 60(3).

Redelmeier, Donald A., and J. Ari Greenwald. 2007. "Competing risks of mortality with marathons: Retrospective analysis." *BMJ* 335: 1275.

Mozaffarian, D., V. L. Roger, et al. 2013. "Heart disease and stroke statis-tics—2013 Update: A report from the American Heart Association." *Circulation* 127(1): e6–e245.

Ornish, D., L. W. Scherwitz, J. H. Billings, et al. 1998. "Intensive lifestyle changes for reversal of coronary heart disease." *JAMA* 280(23): 2001–07.

Fihn, Stephan D., Julius M. Gardin, Jonathan Abrams, Kathleen Berra, James C. Blankenship, et al. 2012. "2012 ACCF/AHA/ACP/AATS/PCNA/SCAI/STS guideline for the diagnosis and management of patients with stable ischemic heart disease." A report of the American College of Cardiology Foundation/American Heart Association Task Force on Practice Guidelines, and the American College of Physicians, American Association for Thoracic Surgery, Preventive Cardiovascular Nurses Association, Society for Cardiovascular Angiography and Interventions, and Society of Thoracic Surgeons. *Circulation* 126: e354–471.

Esselstyn, C. B., Jr. 1999. "Updating a 12-year experience with arrest and reversal therapy for coronary heart disease (an overdue requiem for palliative cardiology)." *Am J Cardiol.* 84: 339–341.

Roger, V.L., A. S. Go, D. M. Lloyd-Jones, et al. 2012. "Heart disease and stroke statistics—2012 update: A report from the American Heart Association." *Circulation* 125(1): e2–220.

Go Red for Women Editors. 2012. "Heart Disease Statistics at a Glance." Accessed at: http://www.goredforwomen.org/about-heart-disease/facts_about_heart_disease_in_women-sub-category/statistics-at-a-glance

Truelsen, Thomas, Stephen Begg, and Colin Mathers. 2000. "The global burden of cerebrovascular disease." Accessed at: http://www.who.int/healthinfo/statistics/bod_cerebrovasculardiseasestroke.pdf

Mackay, J., and G. Mensah. 2004. *The Atlas of Heart Disease and Stroke.* Nonserial publication. World Health Organization. Accessed at: http://www.who.int/cardiovascular_diseases/resources/atlas/en/

Shammas, N. W. 2007. "Epidemiology, classification, and modifiable risk factors of peripheral arterial disease." *Vasc Health Risk Manag.* 3(2): 229–34. doi:10.2147/vhrm.2007.3.2.229. PMC 1994028. PMID 17580733.

Selvin, E., K. Wattanakit, M. W. Steffes, J. Coresh, and A. R. Sharrett. 2006. "HbA1c and peripheral arterial disease in diabetes: The Atherosclerosis Risk in Communities study." *Diabetes Care* 29(4): 877–82. doi:10.2337/diacare.29.04.06.dc05-2018. PMID 16567831.

Jessup, M., W. T. Abraham, D. E. Casey, et al. 2009. "2009 focused update: ACCF/AHA guidelines for the diagnosis and management of heart failure in adults." A report of the American College of Cardiology Foundation/American Heart Association Task Force on Practice Guidelines: developed in collaboration with the International Society for Heart and Lung Transplantation. *Circulation* 119(14): 1977–2016.

Olgin, S. E. 2011. "Approach to the patient with suspected arrhythmia." In L. Goldman and A.I. Schafer, eds. *Cecil Medicine*. 24th ed. Philadelphia, PA: Saunders Elsevier.

Chobanian, A. V., G. L. Bakris, H. R. Black, W. C. Cushman, L. A. Green, J. L. Izzo, Jr., D. W. Jones, et al. 2003. "The Seventh Report of the Joint National Committee on Prevention, Detection, Evaluation, and Treatment of High Blood Pressure: the JNC 7 report." National Heart, Lung, and Blood Institute Joint National Committee on Prevention, Detection, Evaluation, and Treatment of High Blood Pressure; National High Blood Pressure Education Program Coordinating Committee. *JAMA* 289(19): 2560–72.

Centers for Disease Control and Prevention. 2011. "Vital signs: prevalence, treatment, and control of hypertension—United States, 1999–2002 and 2005–2008." *MMWR* 60(4): 103–8.

Institute of Medicine. 2010. *A Population-Based Policy and Systems Change Approach to Prevent and Control Hypertension*. Washington, DC: The National Academies Press. February 22.

Brook, R. D., L. J. Appel, M. Rubenfire, et al. 2013. "Beyond medications and diet: Alternative approaches to lowering blood pressure: A scientific statement from the American Heart Association." *Hypertension*. doi: 10.1161/HYP.0b013e318293645f.

American Diabetes Association. 2011. "Standards of medical care in diabetes—2011." *Diabetes Care* 34 (Suppl. 1): S11–S61.

PubMed Health. 2011. "Type 2 diabetes." Accessed at: http://www.ncbi.nlm.nih.gov/pubmedhealth/PMH0001356/

National Diabetes Information Clearinghouse. (n.d.) "Your guide to diabetes: Type 1 and Type 2."

Forouhi, N. 2006. "The threshold for diagnosing impaired fasting glucose: a position statement by the European Diabetes Epidemiology Group." *Diabetologia* 49:822.

Kim, S. H., L. Chunawala, R. Linde, and G. M. Reaven. 2006. "Comparison of the 1997 and 2003 American Diabetes Association Classification of Impaired Fasting Glucose (IFG): Impact on Prevalence of IFG, Coronary Heart Disease Risk Factors, and Coronary Heart Disease in a Community-Based Medical Practice." *Journal of the American College of Cardiology* 48:293.

Schober S. E., M. D. Carroll, D. A. Lacher, and R. Hirsch. 2007. "High serum total cholesterol—an indicator for monitoring cholesterol lowering efforts; U.S. adults, 2005–2006." NCHS data brief no. 2, Hyattsville, MD: National Center for Health Statistics.

National Institutes of Health. 2001. Third Report of the National Cholesterol Education Program (NCEP) Expert Panel on Detection, Evaluation, and Treatment of High Blood Cholesterol in Adults (Adult Treatment Panel III, or ATP III). Executive summary. *JAMA* 285(19).

Centers for Disease Control and Prevention. 2011. "High blood pressure and cholesterol." *Vital Signs.* Accessed at: http://www.cdc.gov/vitalsigns/pdf/2011-02-vitalsigns.pdf

Daniels, S. R., and F. R. Greer. 2008. "Lipid screening and cardiovascular health in childhood." Committee on Nutrition. *Pediatrics* 122(1):198–208.

U.S. Preventive Services Task Force. 2008. "Screening for lipid disorders in adults." U.S. Preventive Services Task Force recommendation statement. Rockville, MD: Agency for Healthcare Research and Quality.

Brook, Robert D., Lawrence J. Appel, Melvyn Rubenfire, et al. 2013. "Beyond medications and diet: Alternative approaches to lowering blood pressure: A scientific statement from the American Heart Association." *Hypertension* 61: 1360–1383.

Carroll, M. D., B. K. Kit, and D. A. Lacher. 2012. "Total and high-density lipoprotein cholesterol in adults: National Health and Nutrition Examination Survey, 2009–2010." NCHS data brief no. 92. Hyattsville, MD: National Center for Health Statistics.

National Heart, Lung, and Blood Institute. 2012. *Expert Panel on Integrated Guidelines for Cardiovascular Health and Risk Reduction in Children and Adolescents*. NIH Publication No. 12-7486. Accessed at: http://www.nhlbi.nih.gov/guidelines/cvd_ped/peds_guidelines_full.pdf

National Heart, Lung, and Blood Institute. 2011. "What is metabolic syndrome?" Accessed at: http://www.nhlbi.nih.gov/health/health-topics/topics/ms/

American Heart Association. 2012. "What is metabolic syndrome?" Accessed at: http://www.heart.org/idc/groups/heart-public/@wcm/@hcm/documents/downloadable/ucm_300322.pdf

Grundy, Scott M., James I. Cleehan, Stephen R. Daniels, et al. 2005. "Diagnosis and management of the metabolic syndrome: An American Heart Association/National Heart, Lung, and Blood Institute scientific statement." *Circulation* 112: 2735–52.

Aravanis, C., A. Corcondilas, A. S. Dontas, D. Lekos, and A. Keys. 1970. "Coronary heart disease in seven countries." *Circulation* 41 (Suppl. 4): I1–211. PMID 5442782.

Estruch, Ramón, Emilio Ros, Jordi Salas-Salvado, et al. 2013. "Primary prevention of cardiovascular disease with a Mediterranean diet." *New England Journal of Medicine*. doi:10.1056/NEJMoa1200303.

Kolata, Gina. 2013. "Mediterranean diet shown to ward off heart attack and stroke." *New York Times*. February 25.

Slentz, Cris A., Lori B. Aiken, Joseph A. Houmard, Connie W. Bales, Johanna L. Johnson, et al. 2005. "Inactivity, exercise, and visceral fat. STRRIDE: a randomized, controlled study of exercise intensity and amount." *Journal of Applied Physiology* 99(4): 1613–18.

World Cancer Research Fund and American Institute for Cancer Research. 2007. *Food, Nutrition, Physical Activity, and the Prevention of Cancer:*

a Global Perspective. Washington DC: AICR. Accessed at: http://eprints. ucl.ac.uk/4841/1/4841.pdf

World Health Organization. 2003. "WHO/FAO release independent expert report on diet and chronic disease." Accessed at: http://www.who. int/mediacentre/news/releases/2003/pr20/en/

Dawber, Thomas R., Gilcin F. Meadors, and Felix E. Moore, Jr. 1950. *Epidemiological Approaches to Heart Disease: The Framingham Study*. Presented at a Joint Session of the Epidemiology, Health Officers, Medical Care, and Statistics Sections of the American Public Health Association, at the Seventy-eighth Annual Meeting in St. Louis, Mo., November 3, 1950.

O'Donnell, C. J., and R. Elosua. 2008. "Cardiovascular risk factors. Insights from Framingham Heart Study." *Rev Esp Cardiol*. 61(3): 299–310.

Chanh, Tran Tien. 2000. *The Unbalanced Diet Approach to a Slimmer You*. Accessed at: http://www.trantiendiet.com/site/IMG/pdflivre_Dr_Tran.pdf

Freund, K. M., A. J. Belanger, R. B. D'Agostino, and W. B. Kannel. 1993. "The health risks of smoking. The Framingham Study: 34 years of follow-up." *Ann Epidemiol*. 3(4): 417–24.

American Heart Association. 2013. "Smoking & cardiovascular disease (heart disease)." Accessed at: http://www.heart.org/HEARTORG/GettingHealthy/QuitSmoking/QuittingResources/Smoking-Cardiovascular-Disease_UCM_305187_Article.jsp

Chapter 3

Narayan, K. M., J. P. Boyle, T. J. Thompson, S. W. Sorensen SW, and D. F. Williamson. 2003. "Lifetime risk for diabetes mellitus in the United States." *JAMA* 290(14): 1884–90.

Davidson, Michael H., Donald Hunninghake, Kevin C. Maki, Peter O. Kwiterovich, and Stephanie Kafonek. 1999. "Comparison of the effects of lean red meat vs. lean white meat on serum lipid levels among free-living persons with hypercholesterolemia: A long-term, randomized clinical trial." *Arch Intern Med.* 159(12): 1331–38. doi:10.1001/archinte.159.12.1331.

Kimpimäki, T., M. Erkkola, S. Korhonen, A. Kupila, S. M. Virtanen, J. Ilonen, O. Simell, and M. Knip. 2001. "Short-term exclusive breastfeeding predisposes young children with increased genetic risk of type 1 diabetes to progressive beta-cell autoimmunity." *Diabetologia* 44: 63–9.

Dangour, A. D., S. K. Dodhia, A. Hayter, E. Allen, K. Lock, R. Uauy. 2009. "Nutritional quality of organic foods: a systematic review." *American Journal of Clinical Nutrition* 90(3): 680–5.

Smith-Spangler, Crystal, Margaret L. Brandeau, Grace E. Hunter, J. Clay Bavinger, Maren Pearson, Paul J. Eschbach, et al. 2012. "Are organic foods safer or healthier than conventional alternatives? A systematic review." *Ann Intern Med.* 157(5): 348–366.

Brandt, K., C. Leifert, R. Sanderson R, and C. J. Seal. 2011. "Agroecosystem management and nutritional quality of plant foods: The case of organic fruits and vegetables." *Critical Reviews in Plant Sciences* 30: 177–197.

Erdman, J. W., Jr., D. Balentine, L. Arab, et al. 2007. "Flavonoids and heart health: proceedings of the ILSI North America Flavonoids Workshop, May 31–June 1, 2005, Washington, DC." *J Nutr.* 137: 718S–737S.

Huxley, R. R., and H. A. Neil. 2003. "The relation between dietary flavonol intake and coronary heart disease mortality: a meta-analysis of prospective cohort studies." *Eur J Clin Nutr.* 57: 904–908.

Mink, P. J., C. G. Scrafford, L. M. Barraj, et al. 2007. "Flavonoid intake and cardiovascular disease mortality: a prospective study in postmenopausal women." *The American Journal of Clinical Nutrition* 85: 895–909.

Cassidy, A., E. J. O'Reilly, C. Kay, L. Sampson, M. Franz, J. P. Forman, G. Curhan, and E. B. Rimm. 2011. "Habitual intake of flavonoid subclasses and incident hypertension in adults." *The American Journal of Clinical Nutrition* 93: 338–347.

Basu, A., M. Rhone, and T. J. Lyons. 2010. "Berries: emerging impact on cardiovascular health." *Nutr Rev.* 68: 168–177.

Chong, M. F., R. Macdonald, and J. A. Lovegrove. 2010. "Fruit polyphenols and CVD risk: a review of human intervention studies." *The British Journal of Nutrition* 104 (Suppl. 3): S28–39.

Jenkins, D. J., C. W. Kendall, D. G. Popovich, et al. 2001. "Effect of a very-high-fiber vegetable, fruit, and nut diet on serum lipids and colonic function." *Metabolism* 50(4): 494–503.

ScienceDaily. 2011. "Bioactive compounds in berries can reduce high blood pressure." Accessed at: http://www.sciencedaily.com/releases/2011/01/110114155241.htm

Cassidy, A., K. J. Mukamal, L. Liu, M. Franz, A. H. Eliassen, and E. B. Rimm. 2013. "High anthocyanin intake is associated with a reduced risk of myocardial infarction in young and middle-aged women." *Circulation* 127(2): 188–196.

Basu, A., M. Du, M. J. Leyva, et al. 2010. "Blueberries decrease cardiovascular risk factors in obese men and women with metabolic syndrome." *J Nutr.* 140(9): 1582–1587.

Franz, M. J. 2012. "Diabetes mellitus nutrition therapy: Beyond the Glycemic Index: Comment on 'Effect of legumes as part of a low Glycemic Index diet on glycemic control and cardiovascular risk factors in type 2 diabetes mellitus.'" *Arch Intern Med.* 172(21): 1660–1661. doi:10.1001/2013.jamainternmed.871.

Kris-Etherton, P. M., F. B. Hu, E. Ros, and J. Sabate. 2008. "The role of tree nuts and peanuts in the prevention of coronary heart disease: multiple potential mechanisms." *J Nutr.* 138: 1746S–1751S.

Bazzano, L. A., J. He, L. G. Ogden, et al. 2001. "Legume consumption and risk of coronary heart disease in U.S. men and women: NHANES I Epidemiologic Follow-up Study." *Arch Intern Med.* 161(21): 2573–8.

Menotti, A., D. Kromhout, H. Blackburn, F. Fidanza, R. Buzina, and A. Nissinen. 1999. "Food intake patterns and 25-year mortality from coronary heart disease: cross-cultural correlations in the Seven Countries Study. The Seven Countries Study Research Group." *Eur J Epidemiol.* 15(6): 507–15.

Boyle, J. P., T. J. Thompson, E. W. Gregg, L. E. Barker, and D. F. Williamson. 2010. "Projection of the year 2050 burden of diabetes in the US adult population: dynamic modeling of incidence, mortality, and prediabetes prevalence." *Popul Health Metr.* 8(1): 29.

Stolar, M. W. 1988. "Atherosclerosis in diabetes: the role of hyperinsulinemia." *Metabolism* 37(2 Suppl. 1): 1–9.

García, R. G., M. Y. Rincón, W. D. Arenas, et al. 2011. "Hyperinsulinemia is a predictor of new cardiovascular events in Colombian patients with a first myocardial infarction." *Int J Cardiol.* 148(1): 85–90.

Fraser, G. E., J. Sabate, W. L. Beeson, and T. M. Strahan. 1992. "A possible protective effect of nut consumption on risk of coronary heart disease: The Adventist Health study." *Arch Intern Med.* 152(7): 1416–1424.

Griel, A. E., and P. M. Kris-Etherton. 2006. "Tree nuts and the lipid profile: a review of clinical studies." *Br J Nutr.* 96 (Suppl. 2): S68–78.

Nash, S. D., and D. T. Nash. 2008. "Nuts as part of a healthy cardiovascular diet." *Curr Atheroscler Rep.* 10(6): 529–535.

Hites, R. A., J. A. Foran, D. O. Carpenter, M. C. Hamilton, B. A. Knuth, and S. J. Schwager. 2004. "Global assessment of organic contaminants in farmed salmon." *Science* 303(5655): 226–229.

Wongcharoen, Wanwarang, Sasivimon Jai-Aue, Arintaya Phrommintikul, Weerachai Nawarawong, et al. 2012. "Effects of curcuminoids on frequency of acute myocardial infarction after coronary artery bypass grafting." *Am J Cardiol.* 110(1): 40–4.

Akazawa, Nobuhiko, Youngju Choi, Asako Miyaki, Yoko Tanabe, Jun Sugawara, Ryuichi Ajisaka, and Seiji Maeda. "Curcumin ingestion and exercise training improve vascular endothelial function in postmenopausal women." *Nutr Res.* 32(10): 795–9.

Sugawara, Jun, Nobuhiko Akazawa, Asako Miyaki, Youngju Choi, Yoko Tanabe, Tomoko Imai, Seiji Maeda. 2012. "Effect of endurance exercise training and curcumin intake on central arterial hemodynamics in postmenopausal women: Pilot study." *Am J Hypertens.* 25(6): 651–6.

O'Keefe, J. H., K. A. Bybee, and C. J. Lavie. 2007. "Alcohol and cardiovascular health: the razor-sharp double-edged sword." *J Am Coll Cardiol.* 50(11): 1009–14.

Chapter 4

Gibbons, R. J., G. J. Balady, J. W. Beasley, et al. 1997. "ACC/AHA guidelines for exercise testing: executive summary." A report of the American College of Cardiology/American Heart Association Task Force on Practice Guidelines (Committee on Exercise Testing). *J Am Coll Cardiol.* 30: 260–311.

Lynton, H., B. Kligler, and S. Shiflett. 2007. "Yoga in stroke rehabilitation: a systematic review and results of a pilot study." *Top Stroke Rehabil.* 14(4): 1–8.

Bassuk, S. S., and J. E. Manson. 2005. "Epidemiological evidence for the role of physical activity in reducing risk of type 2 diabetes and cardiovascular disease." *J Appl Physiol.* 99(3): 1193–1204.

Duncker, D. J., and R. J. Bache. 2008. "Regulation of coronary blood flow during exercise." *Physiol Rev.* 88(3): 1009–1086.

Verrier, R. L., and A. Tan. 2009. "Heart rate, autonomic markers, and cardiac mortality." *Heart Rhythm* 6: S68–75.

Hamer, M., R. Endrighi, and L. Poole. 2012. "Physical activity, stress reduction, and mood: insight into immunological mechanisms." *Methods Mol Biol.* 934: 89–102.

Hamer, M. 2012. "Psychosocial stress and cardiovascular disease risk: the role of physical activity." *Psychosom Med.* 74(9): 896–903.

Ramsay, L. E., W. W. Yeo, and P. R. Jackson. 1991. "Dietary reduction of serum cholesterol concentration: time to think again." *BMJ* 303(6808): 953–957.

Kojda, G., and R. Hambrecht. 2005. "Molecular mechanisms of vascular adaptations to exercise. Physical activity as an effective antioxidant therapy?" *Cardiovasc Res.* 67(2): 187–197.

Brown, M. D. 2003. "Exercise and coronary vascular remodelling in the healthy heart." *Exp Physiol.* 88(5): 645–658.

Gill, A., R. Womack, and S. Safranek. 2010. "Clinical inquiries: Does exercise alleviate symptoms of depression?" *J Fam Pract.* 59(9): 530–531.

Uebelacker, L. A., G. Epstein-Lubow, B. A. Gaudiano, G. Tremont, C. L. Battle, and I. W. Miller. 2010. "Hatha yoga for depression: critical review of the evidence for efficacy, plausible mechanisms of action, and directions for future research." *J Psychiatr Pract.* 16(1): 22–33.

Saeed, S. A., D. J. Antonacci, and R. M. Bloch. 2010. "Exercise, yoga, and meditation for depressive and anxiety disorders." *Am Fam Physician* 81(8): 981–986.

Atkinson, G., and D. Davenne. 2007. "Relationships between sleep, physical activity and human health." *Physiol Behav.* 90(2–3): 229–235.

Mathur, N., and B. K. Pedersen. 2008. "Exercise as a mean to control low-grade systemic inflammation." *Mediators Inflamm.* Article ID: 109502.

Baldwin, A. L., C. Wagers, A. Towe, and G. E. Schwartz. 2007. "Effects of self-directed reiki and concentration on cutaneous microvascular perfusion of the fingers." *In Focus on Alternative and Complementary Therapies* 12 (Suppl. s1): 6.

Bowden, Deborah, Claire Gaudry, Seung Chan An, and John Gruzelier. 2012. "A Comparative Randomised Controlled Trial of the Effects of Brain Wave Vibration Training, Iyengar Yoga, and Mindfulness on Mood, Well-Being, and Salivary Cortisol." *Evidence-Based Complementary and Alternative Medicine* 2012. Article ID 234713, 13 pages. Doi:10.1155/2012/234713.

Chapter 5

Mathur, N., and B.K. Pedersen. 2008. "Exercise as a mean to control low-grade systemic inflammation." *Mediators Inflamm.* 2008: 109502.

Gill, A., R. Womack, and S. Safranek. 2010. "Clinical Inquiries: Does exercise alleviate symptoms of depression?" *J Fam Pract.* 59: 530–531.

Bhattacharya, A., E. P. McCutcheon, E. Shvartz, and J. E. Greenleaf. 1980. "Body acceleration distribution and O2 uptake in humans during running and jumping." Journal of Applied Physiology 49(5): 881–887.

Richards D. G., D. L. McMillin, E. A. Mein, and C. D. Nelson. 2006. "Colonic irrigations: A review of the historical controversy and the potential for adverse effects." *Journal of Alternative and Complementary Medicine* 12:389–393.

Cider, Åsa, Maria Schaufelberger, Katharina Stibrant Sunnerhagen, and Bert Andersson. 2003. "Hydrotherapy—a new approach to improve function in the older patient with chronic heart failure." Eur J Heart Fail. 5(4): 527–535.

Moffat, Denice M. 2005. Dry Brushing Technique. Accessed at: www.natu-ralhealthtechniques.com/healingtechniquesdry_brushing_technique.htm

Sancier, Kenneth. (n.d.). Anti-Aging Benefits of Qigong. Qigong Institute. Accessed at: http://www.qigonginstitute.org/html/papers/Anti-Aging_Benefits_of_Qigong.html

FX Massage Therapy. 2011. Massage Therapy and Heart Health. Retrieved January 6, 2012, at: http://fxmassage.wordpress.com/2011/02/02/massage-therapy-and-heart-health/

Lee, Y. H., B. N. Park, and S. H. Kim. 2011. "The effects of heat and massage application on autonomic nervous system." Yonsei Medical Journal 52(6): 982–989. Accessed at: http://www.ncbi.nlm.nih.gov/pubmed/22028164

Browne, Richard. 2010. Massage for Heart Health. Acupuncture and Massage College, Inc. Accessed at: http://www.amcollege.edu/acupuncture-massage-blog/massage/massage-for-heart-health/

Rosengren, A., S. Hawken, S. Öunpuu, et al. 2004. "Association of psycho-social risk factors with risk of acute myocardial infarction in 11 119 cases and 13 648 controls from 52 countries (the INTERHEART study): case-control study." Lancet 364: 953–962.

Macleod, J., G. D. Smith, P. Heslop, C. Metcalfe, D. Carroll, and C. Hart. 2002. "Psychological stress and cardiovascular disease: empirical demon-stration of bias in a prospective observational study on Scottish men." BMJ 324: 1247–1251.

Stix, Gary. 2005. "Heavy-metal sweat: Does an infrared sauna really detoxify the body?" Scientific American. October.

Caenar, J. S., J. J. Pflug, N. O. Reig, and L. M. Taylor. 1970. "Lymphatic pressures and the flow of lymph." British Journal of Plastic Surgery 23: 305.

Cunningham, E. 2009. "What impact does pH have on food and nutrition?" *J Am Diet Assoc.* 109(10): 1816. October.

Remer, T. 2000. "Influence of diet on acid-base balance." *Semin Dial.* 13(4): 221–6.

Casa, Douglas J., Priscilla M. Clarkson, and William O. Roberts. 2005. "American College of Sports Medicine Roundtable on Hydration and Physical Activity: Consensus Statements." *Current Sports Medicine Reports* 4:115–127.

Valtzin, H. 2002. "'Drink at least eight glasses of water a day.' Really? Is there scientific evidence for '8 x 8?'" Am J Physiol Regul Integr Comp Physiol. 283: R993–1004.

Rose, B. D., et al. n.d. "Maintenance and replacement fluid therapy in adults." Accessed March 2, 2010, at: http://www.uptodate.com/home/index.html.

Institute of Medicine. 2005. "Dietary Reference Intakes for water, potassium, sodium, chloride, and sulfate." The National Academies Press. Accessed at: http://www.nap.edu/openbook.php?isbn=0309091691

Sawka, M., S. N. Cheuvront, and R. Carter III. 2005. "Human water needs." *Nutrition Reviews* 63:S30–S39.

Manz, F. 2007 "Hydration and disease." *Journal of the American College of Nutritionists* 26(suppl. 5): 535S–541S.

Duyff, R. L. 2012. *American Dietetic Association Complete Food and Nutrition Guide.* 4th ed. Hoboken, NJ: John Wiley & Sons. 159.

Bibbins-Domingo, K., G. M. Chertow, P. G. Coxson, A. Moran, J. M. Lightwood, M. J. Pletcher, and L. Goldman. 2010. "Projected effect of dietary salt reductions on future cardiovascular disease." *New England Journal of Medicine* 362:590.

Sheps, S. G. (ed.). 2008. *Mayo Clinic: 5 Steps to Controlling High Blood Pressure.* Rochester, MN: Mayo Foundation for Medical Education and Research.

Harvard Medical School. 2006. "The truth about fats: bad and good." Family Health Guide. Accessed at: http://www.health.harvard.edu/fhg/updates/Truth-about-fats.shtml

Howard, Barbara V., and Judith Wylie-Rosett. 2002. "Sugar and cardiovascular disease: a statement for healthcare professionals from the Committee on Nutrition of the Council on Nutrition, Physical Activity, and Metabolism of the American Heart Association." Circulation 106: 523–527.

Archer S. L., K. Liu, A. R. Dyer, K. J. Ruth, D. R. Jacobs, Jr., L. Van Horn, J. E. Hilner, and P. J. Savage. 1998. "Relationship between changes in dietary sucrose and high density lipoprotein cholesterol: the CARDIA study. Coronary Artery Risk Development in Young Adults. Ann Epidemiol. 8(7): 433–8.

Duke Medicine News and Communications. 2002. "Caffeine's effects are long-lasting and compound stress." DukeHealth.org. National Institutes of Health July/August 2002 issue of *Psychosomatic Medicine.* Accessed at: http://www.dukehealth.org/health_library/news/5687

Science Blog. 2004. "Highlights of the NIAAA position paper on moderate alcohol consumption." June. Alcoholism: Clinical and Experimental Research. Accessed at: http://scienceblog.com/community/older/2004/1/2004232.shtml

Chapter 6

Woollard, M., J. Poposki, B. McWhinnie, L. Rawlins, G. Munro, and P. O'Meara. 2011. "Achy breaky makey wakey heart? A randomised crossover trial of musical prompts." Emergency Medicine Journal 29: 290–294. DOI: 10.1136/emermed-2011-200187.

Carnethon, M., L. P. Whitsel, B. A. Franklin, P. Kris-Etherton, R. Milani, C. A. Pratt, and G. R. Wagner. 2009. "Worksite wellness programs for cardiovascular disease prevention: a policy statement." *Circulation* 120: 1725–1741. Print ISSN: 0009-7322. Online ISSN: 1524-4539.

Better Health Channel. 2013. "Health benefits of dancing." Dance-health benefits. Accessed at: http://www.betterhealth.vic.gov.au/bhcv2/bhcarticles.nsf/pages/Dance_health_benefits

Verghese, J., R. B. Lipton, M. J. Katz, C. B. Hall, C. A. Derby, G. Kuslansky, A. F. Ambrose, M. Sliwinski, and H. Buschke. 2003. "Leisure activities and the risk of dementia in the elderly." *N Engl J Med*. 348: 2508–2516. June 19, 2003.

Bittman, B. B., L. S. Berk, D. L. Felten, J. Westengard, O. C. Simonton, J. Pappas, and M. Ninehouser. 2001. "Reversal of the hormonal stress response and an increase in natural killer cell activity (an enhanced immune system) in blood samples from participants in an hour-long drumming session." *Alternative Therapies* (7)1.

Friedman, R. L. 1994. "A reduction in anxiety and distress and an increase in self-esteem in a study of 30 depressed people over 80 years of age who participated in weekly drumming/music therapy sessions at Stanford University School of Medicine." *The Healing Power of the Drum*.

Marano, H. E. 2003. "The benefits of laughter." Psychology Today. Accessed at: http://www.psychologytoday.com/articles/200304/the-benefits-laughter

Cousins, N. 1976. "Anatomy of an illness as perceived by the patient. N Engl J Med. 295(26): 1458–63. Accessed at http://www.PubMed.gov

Devereux, P. G., and K. L. Heffner. 2007. "Psychophysiological approaches to the study of laughter: toward an integration with positive psychology." In A. D. Ong and M. van Dulmen (eds.), *Oxford Handbook of Methods in Positive Psychology*. New York, NY: Oxford University Press. pp. 233–49.

Martin, R. A. 2001. "Humor, laughter, and physical health: methodological issues and research findings." Psychol Bull. 127(4): 504–19. Accessed at: http://www.PubMed.gov

Martin, R. A. 2002. "Is laughter the best medicine? Humor, laughter, and physical health." *Curr Dir Psychol Sci.*11(6):216–20.

Babauta, L. 2009. "The 10 essential rules for slowing down and enjoying life more." Zenhabits. Accessed at: http://zenhabits.net/the-10-essential-rules-for-slowing-down-and-enjoying-life-more/

Chapter 7

National Heart Lung and Blood Institute. 2005. "Your Guide to Living Well with Heart Disease." Accessed at: http://www.nhlbi.nih.gov/health/public/heart/other/your_guide/living_well.pdf

Womenshealth.gov. 2009. "Heart Health and Stroke." Accessed at: http://www.womenshealth.gov/heart-health-stroke/

American Heart Association. 2012. "Stress and Heart Health." Accessed at: http://www.heart.org/HEARTORG/Conditions/More/MyHeartand-StrokeNews/Stress-and-Heart-Health_UCM_437370_Article.jsp

McCarty, R., G. Aguilera, E. L. Sabban, and R. Kvetnansky. 2002. *Stress: Neural, Endocrine, and Molecular Studies.* CRC Press.

Barbor, C. 2001. "The science of meditation." Psychology Today. Accessed at: http://www.psychologytoday.com/articles/200105/the-science-meditation

Murphy, M., S. Donovan, and E. Taylor. 1997. *The Physical and Psychological Effects of Meditation: A Review of Contemporary Research with a Comprehensive Bibliography, 1931–1996.* Institute of Noetic Sciences; Subsequent edition (June 1997).

Kok, Bethany E., Kimberly A. Coffey, Michael A. Cohn, Lahnna I. Catalino Tanya Vacharkulksemsuk, Sara B. Algoe, Mary Brantley, and Barbara

L. Fredrickson, 2013. "How Positive Emotions Build Physical Health." *Psychological Science 24 (7)* 1123-1132.

Schmidt, T. F. H., A. H. Wijga, B. P. Robra, M. J. Muller, et al. 1995. "Yoga training and vegetarian nutrition reduce cardiovascular risk factors in healthy Europeans." *Homeostasis in Health and Disease* 36:66.

Agarwal, B. L., and A. Kharbanda. 1990. "Effect of transcendental meditation on mild and moderate hypertension." In R. A. Chalmers, G. Schenkluhn, et al. (eds.), *Scientific Research on Maharishi's Transcendental Meditation and TM-Sidhi Programme: Collected Papers.* Vol. 3.

Zeidan, F., K. T. Martucci, R. A. Kraft, J. G. McHaffie, and R. C. Coghill. 2013. "Neural correlates of mindfulness meditation-related anxiety relief." *Social Cognitive and Affective Neuroscience.*

Fernros, L., A.-K. Furhoff, and P. E. Wandell. 2008. "Improving quality of life using compound mind-body therapies: evaluation of a course intervention with body movement and breath therapy, guided imagery, chakra experiencing and mindfulness meditation." *Quality of Life Research* 17: 367–376.

Sandor, M. K. 2005. "The labyrinth: a walking meditation for healing and self-care." *Explore* (New York, NY) 1:480–483.

Dusek, J. A., P. L. Hibberd, B. Buczynski, B. H. Chang, K. C. Dusek, J. M. Johnston, A. L. Wohlhueter, H. Benson, and R. M. Zusman. 2008. "Stress management versus lifestyle modification on systolic hypertension and medication elimination: a randomized trial." *Journal of Alternative and Complementary Medicine* 14: 129–138.

Kennerly, R. 2004. "QEEG analysis of binaural beat audio entrainment: a pilot study." *Journal of Neurotherapy* 8(2): 122.

Lane, J., S. Kasian, J. Owens, and G. Marsh. 1998. "Binaural auditory beats affect vigilance performance and mood." *Physiology & Behavior* 63(2): 249–252.

Green, E. E., and A. M. Green. 1986. "Biofeedback and states of consciousness." In B. B. Wolman and M. Ullman (eds.), *Handbook of States of Consciousness*. New York: Van Nostrand Reinhold.

Hutchison, M. 1990. "Special issue on sound/light." *Megabrain Report* 1(2).

Mavromatis, A. 1987. *Hypnagogia: The Unique State of Consciousness Between Wakefulness and Sleep*. New York: Routledge & Kegan Paul.

Richardson, A., and F. McAndrew. 1990. "The effects of photic stimulation and private self-consciousness on the complexity of visual imagination imagery." *British Journal of Psychology* 81: 381–394.

Rossi, E. L. 1986. *The Psychobiology of Mind-Body Healing*. New York: W. W. Norton.

Garland, Eric, and Matthew Owen Howard. 2009. "Neuroplasticity, psychosocial genomics, and the biopsychosocial paradigm in the 21st century." *Health Soc Work.* 34(3): 191–199.

Huang, Tina, and Christine Charyton. 2008. "A comprehensive review of the psychological effects of brainwave entrainment." *Alternative Therapies in Health and Medicine* 14(5).

Middlekauff, H. R., K. Hui, J. L. Yu, M. A. Hamilton, G. C. Fonarow, J. Moriguchi, W. R. Maclellan, and A. Hage. 2002. "Acupuncture inhibits sympathetic activation during mental stress in advanced heart failure patients." *J Card Fail.* 8(6):399–406.

Shiina, Yumi, Nobusada Funabashi, Kwangho Lee, Tomohiko Toyoda, Tai Sekine, Sachiko Honjo, et al. 2008. "Relaxation effects of lavender aromatherapy improve coronary flow velocity reserve in healthy men evaluated by transthoracic Doppler Echocardiogram." *Int J Cardiol.* 129 (2):193–7.

Lee, C. O. 2003. "Clinical aromatherapy, Part II: Safe guidelines for integration into clinical practice." *Clin J Oncol Nurs.* 7(5):597–8.

Dinsha, Darius. 1996. *Let There Be Light.* Dinshah Health Society; 4th edition (June).

Christian, Caitlin. Crystal Therapy. Vanderbilt University Health Psychology. Accessed at: http://healthpsych.psy.vanderbilt.edu/crystal_healing.htm

Rindge, David. 2007. "Laser therapy and cardiovascular disease." Acupuncture Today. April.

Lieverse, Ritsaert; Eus J. W. Van Someren, Marjan M. A. Nielen, Bernard M. J. Uitdehaag, Jan H. Smit, and Witte J. G. Hoogendijk. 2011. "Bright light treatment in elderly patients with nonseasonal Major Depressive Disorder." *Arch Gen Psychiatry.* 68(1):61–70. doi:10.1001/archgenpsychiatry.2010.183.

Aldridge, David. 1996. *Music Therapy Research and Practice in Medicine from Out of the Silence.* Jessica Kingsley.

Donaldson, F. O. 1993. *Playing by Heart: The vision and practice of belonging.* Deerfield Beach, FL: Health Communications, Inc.

Thompson, J. F., and P. C. Kam. 1995. "Music in the operating theatre." British Journal of Surgery 82:12. 1586–1587. Accessed at http://www.pain.com/painscripts/Pain Search.dll?2

Bradt, Joke, and Cheryl Dileo. 2009. "Music for stress and anxiety reduction in coronary heart disease patients." Published online: 15 April. Assessed as up to date: 10 October 2008. DOI: 10.1002/14651858. CD006577.pub2.

Friedman, Rachel S. C., Matthew M. Burg, Pamela Miles, Forrester Lee, and Rachel Lampert. 2010. "Effects of reiki on autonomic activity early after acute coronary syndrome." *J. Am. Coll. Cardiol.* 56: 995–996.

Chapter 8

Smith, Calvin Dale. (n.d.). Internal Causes of Disease: Emotional Dishar-mony. Riverside Acupuncture and Wellness Centre. Accessed at: http://www.calvindale.com/disease.html

Cohen, Ken. 1999. *The Way of Qigong: The Art and Science of Chinese Energy Healing.* Wellspring/Ballantine; 1 edition. March 9.

Gruber, June, Iris B. Mauss, and Maya Tamir. 2011. "A dark side of happi-ness? How, when and why happiness is not always good." *Perspectives on Psychological Science* 6(3): 222–233.

LaBerge, Stephen. 2000. "Lucid dreaming: Evidence that REM sleep can support unimpaired cognitive function and a powerful methodology for studying the psychophysiology of dreaming." Behavioral and Brain Sciences 23(6): 962–963.

CREDITS

The following are the intellectual properties of the authors listed below and have been reproduced with permission in writing by the copyright holders:

Figure 1-1

Images taken from Cardiac Chamber Formation: Development, Genes, and Evolution, Copyright 2003 by Dr. Antoon F. M. Moorman.

Figure 1-2

Copyright alila/123RF

Figure 2-1

Copyright Peter Junaidy/123RF

Figure 3-1, 3-2

Copyright Nutrition Security Institute

Figure 3-3, 3-4

Images taken from *Eat For Health*, Copyright 2008, 2012 by Joel Fuhrman, M.D.

Figure 7-1

Copyright 2012 The Tapping Solution, LLC